MW01014141

the
CODE

the
CODe

Unlocking the Ancient Power of Your Birthday

Johanna Paungger / Thomas Poppe

ATRIA BOOKS
New York London Toronto Sydney

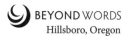
BEYOND WORDS
Hillsboro, Oregon

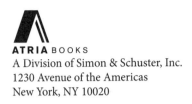

ATRIA BOOKS
A Division of Simon & Schuster, Inc.
1230 Avenue of the Americas
New York, NY 10020

BEYOND WORDS
20827 N.W. Cornell Road, Suite 500
Hillsboro, Oregon 97124-9808
503-531-8700 / 503-531-8773 fax
www.beyondword.com

Managing editor: Lindsay S. Brown
Editor: Julie Steigerwaldt
Copyeditor: Henry Covey
Proofreader: Jennifer Weaver-Neist
Design: Devon Smith
Composition: William H. Brunson Typography Services

First Atria Books/Beyond Words hardcover edition September 2011

ATRIA BOOKS and colophon are trademarks of Simon & Schuster, Inc.
Beyond Words Publishing is a division of Simon & Schuster, Inc.

For more information about special discounts for bulk purchases,
please contact Simon & Schuster Special Sales at 1-866-506-1949 or
business@simonandschuster.com.

The Simon & Schuster Speakers Bureau can bring authors to your live event.
For more information or to book an event, contact the Simon & Schuster Speakers
Bureau at 1-866-248-3049 or visit our website at www.simonspeakers.com.

Manufactured in China

10 9 8 7 6 5 4 3 2 1

Library of Congress Cataloging-in-Publication Data
Paungger, Johanna.
  [Tiroler Zahlenrad. English]
    The code : unlocking the ancient power of your birthday / Johanna Paungger,
  Thomas Poppe. — 1st Atria Books/Beyond Words hardcover ed.
      p. cm.
  1. Fortune-telling by birthdays. I. Poppe, Thomas. II. Title.
  BF1891.B54P38 2011
  133.3'354—dc22
                                                            2011005555
  ISBN: 978-1-58270-289-6
  ISBN: 978-1-4516-1281-3 (ebook)

The corporate mission of Beyond Words Publishing, Inc.: *Inspire to Integrity*

Contents

We are thankful to the East because everyone feels good in the morning when they awake,
And see the bright light coming from the East,
And when the Sun goes down in the West, we feel good and glad we are well;
Then we are thankful to the West.
And we are thankful to the North, because when the cold winds come
We are glad to have lived to see the leaves fall again;
And to the South, for when the south wind blows
And everything is coming up in the spring,
We are glad to live to see the grass growing and everything green again.
We thank the Thunders, for they are the Mani'towuk that bring the rain,
Which the Creator has given them power to rule over.
And we thank our mother, the Earth.

—From *Religion and Ceremonies of the Lenape*
by M. R. Harrington

Note from the Editor

I am pleased to introduce to you *The Code*, by Johanna Paungger and Thomas Poppe, now available to English readers for the first time. *The Code* is different from anything I have come across before, going far beyond other numerology books and similar systems. It is authentic indigenous knowledge passed down through generations and as such is part of a much larger ancient healing tradition. It combines two dimensions working together: the power of one's birthdate and the energies of colors. And it uses the Birthday Wheel, which has energetic motion and the points of the compass—North, East, South, West, and Center—as do symbols from many other ancient traditions, such as the Native American medicine wheel.

Most important, *The Code* is not just about who we are but about who we can be; this is a system that people can use to better guide their life and fulfill their true potential. It opens the door to living life in a more harmonious and peaceful way, in tune with our own gifts.

People continue to be curious about their unique self and also want to know more about the people in their lives: friends, family, loved ones, and co-workers. They want tools that will empower them, and for this reason, the wisdom contained here is something that I know readers will be keenly interested in. By combining the Numbers and colors on the Number Wheel, we get to see the picture of the person as a whole. If you want to understand your children better; find out why your partner or spouse reacts as she or he does; improve your relationships at home or at work; develop your social, artistic, and monetary skills; or if you have always wondered about the attitudes of your friends or co-workers, you will find the answers in *The Code*!

I have seen for myself that the system works by using it in my own life. Because there is more to it than just the right Numbers, I have surrounded myself with the colors that complement my Signature, or personalized Code. I've edited my closet to the recommended colors and the specific tasks I face. For example, when the situation calls for organization and efficiency, I wear white. I can feel the difference. Not only do I get more things done wearing white, I get more compliments as well—which, by the way, has also simplified shopping and picking out what to wear! These steps may seem simple, but they make an impact.

The Code has taken off in the Beyond Words office, too. People have written Numbers on circles cut out of appropriately colored Post-it notes and stuck them to their computers. There are conversations about balancing out missing Cardinal Points (compass directions) and Numbers. And new colors have been showing up in many other wardrobes as well.

The Code resonates for many different people for many different reasons. One of the ways that it resonated for me was the fact that it fits into the unusual category of *indigenous* Western knowledge (Celtic, Norse, and so on). Western readers come from all over, and many can trace their heritage to Europe, where Johanna's family's knowledge originated. This book returns to those ancestral roots. As Westerners, our ancestors likely lived their lives in tune with this wisdom. We have simply lost touch with it, and now is our opportunity to restore the connection.

The authors, Johanna and Thomas, are an absolute delight, and their great passion for this ancient knowledge is part of who they are. *The Code* was kept silent for generations, and their desire to share it with the world for the benefit of all is genuine. They do not proselytize or try to convince;

they simply know their knowledge works and offer it to us should we choose to use it.

And many people do. The authors have been bestsellers in Europe for over twenty years. They have written books on topics such as our connection to nature, the lunar cycle, diet, and biorhythms—books which have sold more than fourteen million copies in twenty-four languages. In Europe, many doctors and dentists consult Johanna and Thomas's books before scheduling surgery or other procedures. Organic farmers look to them before planting, harvesting, and performing many of their key tasks. The authors' knowledge of moon timing is used by the general public to create better outcomes in many areas such as healing, gardening, construction, running a household, and daily living, just to name a few. We couldn't be more delighted to help make their message available to an even wider audience.

The Code offers a key for opening up the lost treasures and talents hidden deep within us. It provides a guide to relationships, work, health, and living a fulfilling life. *The Code* unfolds from the rhythms of nature and as such can bring harmony, balance, and a deeper connection with others and the world around us. It does all of this and more, and is very easy to learn and use.

Thomas and Johanna have many more books on the Number system, Moon Timing, Lunar Calendar Lore, and other ancestral wisdom that they are ready to share with us. We feel that this book is the perfect introduction because it offers a window into their worldview and gives a hint of what to expect in their forthcoming books. We hope you'll enjoy *The Code* and stay tuned for what's to come.

Cynthia Black

Cynthia Black, Editor in Chief
Beyond Words Publishing, Inc.

Growing Up with the Code

Johanna Paungger

In this book, I would like to introduce you to a very special chapter from my early years on my family's mountain farm in the Austrian Alps. It was there that I learned about the ancient knowledge that centers on the far-reaching and significant influence of one's date of birth. This special combination of Numbers—the month, day, and year in which you were born—contains a hidden treasure that you can unearth with the help of this book. It is much like being given the combination to a safe, the contents of which only you can access.

When I observe what's going on in the world today, I see signs that many people are now willing and able to return to the time-honored knowledge of our ancestors, which makes me very happy. Anyone—in any walk of life—can benefit from this knowledge, and this readiness around the globe makes it the perfect time to disclose the secret of the Code.

Unspoken Family Wisdom

The farm on which I lived until I was fifteen was bought by my grandfather Joseph in the 1930s. He succeeded a family who had lived there generation after generation for over two hundred years. Located in the Tyrol area of western Austria, the farm was big enough to house all our family members: my grandfathers, grandmothers, parents, nine siblings, foster children, cousins, and farm hands. We were a lively crowd and dedicated stewards to working the little plot of flora and fauna under our care.

Observing the cycles and rhythms of nature, we knew without a shadow of doubt that the forests, meadows, fields, waterways, and wells in our care were not to be exploited for human consumption but cared for harmoniously. Everybody in our home was integrated into everyday life on the farm and worked until about the age of eighteen. Then came the time to move on with one's own life and follow a calling, either by marrying or setting up a business as a baker, carpenter, or engineer.

We had everything a farm was supposed to have—cornfields, fruit trees, animals, herb gardens, forests—and we tended all of it without artificial fertilizers or pesticides. The steep terrains we worked with horses or with our bare hands. We knew how to accept and manage pests and blights, which we never thought of as such. Pest and blight are mere words in the sentences of the language that nature uses to speak to us. We listened, and then we did the right thing to accept and manage the so-called problems. The modern style of violently battling symptoms instead of looking for real causes was never our style.

Looking back at our everyday life, I realize that it was, in many ways, very different from what is regarded as normal today, even by the standards of Tyrolean farmers. For example, when it came to living by the Code, my family had nothing in writing about it and no formal teaching about its use. Although we knew that the Code worked, we did not know why it worked. We lived by this special knowledge of Birthday Numbers and benefited from it, but we did not probe deeper. Instead, we took it for granted, just as we took the seasons for granted or the fact that thunder followed lightning. The Numbers became part of our flesh and blood. It would have felt strange and crazy not to use them, just as it would have felt crazy to take a pill to battle a headache instead of treating the cause.

The Code was effective and valuable, and we incorporated it without question, without talking about it. I have since discovered that merely a handful of people outside of my family were aware of the Code's existence—far fewer than I had thought. Although many of the people who came to my grandfather for help greatly benefited from the Code, no one had an inkling of its existence.

My grandfather was an unpretentious farmer with an exceptional amount of knowledge about all the facets of human nature. The fact that he was deaf most certainly helped him understand people better. When I was at a loss comprehending people's actions and motives, he always used to tell me to cover my ears by pressing my palms against them. As a child, this instantly brought me in contact with my inner voice—my intuitive perception, as I would call it today. I can always trust that voice; everybody can. But most of us have been bribed away from that way of perceiving reality. Fortunately, it is never too late to turn inward again.

When grandfather and I went on long hikes together (which I did from the age of three onward), I saw that animals, humans, rocks, herbs, and water formed a unified whole and that only our thought processes created the split between them. We always found the healing herb that was meant for a specific person at a specific time, because the herb made itself felt— as if it talked to us. Then we either used it right away, or it was dried and stored for later. And that future moment of necessity almost always came.

Grandfather dedicated his whole life to family, nature, and healing people. Because I cried a lot as a baby and because he was deaf, my crib was set up in his room—at which point, I immediately stopped crying. Since I lived in his room from almost day one, I learned many things in those younger years, knowing that whatever he taught was important. He never had to justify himself to me (as was sometimes the case with patients). His teaching was really a kind of assimilation without words. Once, I overheard him tell his brother that he never noticed his deafness when he was on our usual long walks with me. He didn't miss a thing then. And I never felt his deafness was an impediment in communicating with him. We had a kind of telepathic rapport, which lasted until his death.

Grandfather's specialty as a shaman and healer was complete removal of others' pain. He was a master at it, and people came from far and wide to be healed, even in the most serious cases. Many doctors and physicians came to us with their families as well. His repertoire combined extensive herbal knowledge with the ancient arts of healing in harmony with the lunar calendar, healthy nutrition, and of course, the Code. When asked to recommend a course of action, he often told people what to let go of, whether it be a habit, food, or activity. What *not* to do was and is, in most cases, the road to true healing. Maybe that's why the most truly fulfilling accomplishments in life feel as if no effort was necessary.

My earliest memories of working with the Code are rather vague. I do remember, however, that I knew the Numbers before I started school. Although I doubt that I was aware of their deeper meaning, I remember drawing certain Numbers on colored slips of paper for my grandfather. Sometimes, when a difficult task lay ahead or something required a great deal of energy, we were given those Numbers on the colored paper to help us with our particular task. But it was done inconspicuously, so as not to attract attention. Even as children, my siblings and I intuitively sensed that the use of this knowledge was not to be discussed.

How We Used the Code

As a true healer, my grandfather used the Code as part of his vast treasure of treatments and methods. He had the ability to recognize a problem's underlying cause and heal it. For him, a physical symptom was merely a marker pointing to the root of the problem. For that very reason, he treated each person on an individual basis. Although two people may have appeared to have identical symptoms, they rarely received the same treatment. My grandfather used the Code primarily to better understand that person, especially if he or she was extremely stubborn or had little faith in my grandfather's alternative healing methods. Fortunately, he had infinite patience with such people and was always determined to do what was needed to help them.

In my family, the Numbers were also helpful when dealing with other children—and there were lots. Our parents and grandparents usually paid close attention to our individual Numbers, assigning daily chores and larger tasks accordingly. Most of the time this made sense, and the results showed it.

Yet, seen through the eyes of a child, there were also disadvantages to this approach. According to my personal Numbers, I was able to do chores independently and responsibly, and as such, was expected to. Sometimes, I would have liked the chance to enjoy the very things that I did not seem to need: a little more attention, support, and teamwork. I learned the hard way that drawing upon the wisdom of the Code can result in expecting too much from a child who has a certain Number combination.

I was not alone in that; some of my siblings felt the same way. And at times, this was difficult for us. However, when I was growing up, such things were not discussed. Fortunately, life provides the opportunity to make up for many things in our past. In the course of time, I learned this lesson: the best way to heal is to not saddle our children with the same burden. Almost any hurt we suffered as children can be healed by not repeating the same mistake when raising our own children. This is a law of nature.

The Code was also helpful when dealing with other children, especially when we had to babysit our neighbors' kids. By finding out the dates of birth of those put in our charge, we would know ahead of time what it would take for the little ones to fall into a deep slumber. For example, children with certain Numbers should be told soothing stories, while children with other Numbers should be allowed to run around before bedtime. We also consulted the Code when it came to picking the color of their pajamas and bedding. For me, the clearest proof of the Code's effectiveness came from watching these children's behavior.

The Right Timing

People sometimes ask, "If you knew of the Numbers your whole life, why did you wait until now to publish the Code?" I had originally planned to publish at the beginning of the year 2000 because of the special energy of the ❷ and the ⓪ in the digits of the second millennium. The new Numbers promised a new openness toward this type of information, where people would be more receptive to ideas that truly worked without needing the approval of the scientific community. A number of events, however, soon made my husband, Thomas, and I realize that the time was not yet ripe.

In a time of total technological addiction and widespread conviction that evil and terror could be eradicated through fighting instead of understanding, there was no room for this kind of knowledge in the past decade. Imagine someone who is absolutely convinced that cancer can be cured by chemotherapy and radiation. Then tell this person that he just needs to change his way of thinking and his diet to remove the real cause of his ailment. Now you have an idea why we had to postpone publication.

Today, this viewpoint is changing, and people worldwide are willing to consider that imagined security is no security at all. There is a new willingness to absorb the kind of material contained in our books and messages. The ancient knowledge of the Code is too valuable to become just another fad. And as the caretaker of this knowledge, I have a responsibility and an obligation to guard it. Everything has its time, and short-term thinking rarely makes for good timing.

The second reason for my discretion is that because this nature-based system evolved from farmers, I did not want to compromise their social standing in a culture where science and statistics are revered over intuition and natural rhythms. Farmers in a rural community typically have little support, while churches, school principals, mayors, and physicians hold all the authority. At times, I think that farming evolved into a science-driven, nature-exploiting industry in order to move farmers up in the social pecking order.

Organic farmers, who live and work in harmony with nature, deserve our greatest respect. They keep us connected to nature through ancient wisdom and philosophies, contribute to a sustainable future, and help us stay healthy by providing genuine food for our table. Unfortunately, in the eyes of some, they remain "only" farmers.

Over centuries, this low standing within an artificially created social network led farmers to develop special survival skills, and the result was the practicality and "peasant's cunning" for which farmers are so well known. One of the basic elements of these strategies was recognizing a child's potential at an early age, which is simple when using the Code. The Code was actually part of a secret defense mechanism for people who, over centuries, were subject to various forms of exploitation and suppression.

Maintaining utmost secrecy about most things was a natural component of this survival strategy. This also applied to the Code. Unlike today, children were not allowed to speak up around adults when I was growing up. Rather, children were supposed to speak only when spoken to. It was unheard of, especially for us girls, to discuss problems, chatter endlessly, interrupt a conversation, or have a conversation on an equal basis with our parents. Fortunately, times have changed.

I do, however, become pensive occasionally when I see what is considered normal today. As I look back on my childhood and our family life, I think that much of the old knowledge would have quickly disappeared had current forms of communication been available during that time. *After all, what happens to observation skills when anything can be asked at any time?* If, as a child, I am satisfied with the answers of adults and my knowledge comes strictly from books and the internet, an entire world is lost.

This, in an indirect way, is how I came to learn about the Code—by watching, imitating, and putting faith into it. Mainly, I listened and, if necessary, eavesdropped when the grown-ups were talking. Today, I know that knowledge obtained from observing and listening is retained far better than anything taught by traditional methods in school.

My grandparents and parents were secretive about the Code, but if you read between the lines of what was said, you could pick up certain messages. One of these messages was especially emphatic: "The Church is against it!" That was the third reason why Thomas and I waited so long to publish this book. The Catholic Church has historically been against any practice that resembles paganism, even though the Church has frequently conducted pagan rites over the centuries. You would be hard-pressed to find a pulpit in historic churches that had not been carefully positioned by using a dowsing rod or a pendulum. Wherever a church or sect is concerned with power and glory instead of true faith, it finds a way to oppose and devalue anything that might lead its flock to emotional and intellectual independence. For that very reason, institutions monopolized esoteric knowledge, like dowsing, consulting the pendulum, the art of lunar timing, herbal and mystical remedies, as well as many, many other aids that helped people cope with their daily lives. Under no circumstances was this knowledge to be used without the blessing of established authorities, and that's why my family feared sharing the Code.

As such, the Code was, in a sense, a secret practice that was not even discussed among siblings. During our last get-together a few years ago, I mentioned to my brothers and sisters that I wanted to publish this knowledge. Their reaction ranged from shock to benevolent understanding. Even now, I feel somewhat uneasy about passing it on. But I confronted my fears and realized that they were unwarranted. It would have been far more damaging to keep this secret hidden.

The knowledge revealed in this book can pave the way to a more fair and healthy world. Recognizing one's strengths and weaknesses becomes much easier with its help. The Code can be instrumental in counteracting, supporting, or promoting important events and energies. From unemployment offices to human resource personnel, from schoolteachers to shamans, from physicians to holistic healers, from all the children of the world to all its senior citizens—the list of who can benefit is endless.

The Code can provide as much help for us now as it did in my childhood. You will have an instrument that helps you to take charge of your life and assume responsibility for it in all its facets and colors. This kind of responsibility is not a burden but part of a joyously accepted and practiced birthright. Use the Code carefully, wisely, and with respect, and you will find a new, friendlier world. You will see with different eyes into a brighter future.

The Hidden Birthday Present

Thomas Poppe

The Code is a hidden gem emerging from nature's unspoken truths, and I am certain of one thing: it can be a great help in anything—from thoughtful child rearing to choosing a career based upon genuine but still-hidden talents. It can contribute to sensible, preventive healthcare, targeted healing, and symptom relief. This book will help you get to know yourself much better; your strengths, your weaknesses, and maybe even your hidden talents will become more apparent to you. After reading this book and using the Code, you may even experience a feeling of relief, as though a heavy fog and numbness have lifted.

In its place, you will develop the courage to look beyond the obvious, make a fresh start, and get rid of old baggage. Our hope is that this book will bring about the turning point you have been searching for, consciously or unconsciously. Many of us are unhappy in our current situation or have the feeling that we are living in the wrong place at the wrong time, that our real life is still waiting for us, or, worse, that we have missed our opportunity. You can change that by using this book. It is never too late to make a fresh start.

I started this journey with the Code many years ago, when I met Johanna and she slowly began to reveal some elements of its wisdom as it became apparent that I would treat it responsibly. For nearly twenty years, we shared almost everything else—our home and our workspace, the writing of seven books, the design of eight calendars, and the happy parenting of three kids; the Code was the exception. All the while, I was unaware of the Code working in Johanna's daily routines, though her uncanny ability to remember hundreds of birthdays struck me as unusual. She simply saw a birthdate in full color and in three dimensions in her mind's eye. Then one day, almost overnight, the basic structure of the Code emerged, and after long, long talks, she revealed what people's dates of birth told her about them. What a treasure!

It was only until recently that I (gently) convinced Johanna, after consulting with her siblings, to unearth and share with others this treasure from her family's fount of secret, ancient knowledge. Convincing her was not easy, for the very reasons Johanna discussed in the previous pages, and made it equally challenging to document the carefully guarded knowledge of the Code.

When Johanna talks about the secrecy in her family and the silence that surrounded the Code, I am reminded of a family get-together shortly before we started working on this book. At that time, we had already decided to publish *The Code*, so I was looking forward to talking with Johanna's sisters and brothers in the hope of gaining a more complete understanding. I had known them all for many years and was looking forward to soaking up every tidbit of information possible for the book. And Johanna encouraged me to do so, because she was not sure she could remember everything.

As it turned out, it was a lost labor of love, but not because of Johanna's family's ill will. They all told me quite convincingly that they had no recall of the Code. Just a few minutes later, however, after I had unsuccessfully questioned the most reliable source among Johanna's siblings, this very sister casually commented on the artistic abilities of one of her nieces by saying matter-of-factly, "No wonder, with those Numbers." My response was immediate. "So you do know after all?" Her solemn and honest answer came just as quickly as her last statement about the Numbers of her niece:

"Oh no, I really have no idea." From then on, I refrained from asking further questions.

This experience did not really come as a surprise. When interacting with Johanna's family, I learned early on that much of the communication went on below the surface. Whenever they all got together, I was surprised by how my wife and her siblings seemed to communicate with the unfailing surety of honeybees. It was as if they could read each other's minds. Their glances, little gestures, and certain catchwords all painted a picture of overall harmony—even at times when there was tension in the air. It felt like I was attending a meeting of a secret society in which all its members were able to turn base metal into gold except me.

After lengthy conversations with Johanna, I gradually began to understand just what was behind this behavior. You see, where Johanna grew up, country folk were almost always silent when the city folk were talking. When farmers did speak, they did so in their rural country dialect. As a result, the urbanites and academics thought the farmers were just "dumb." To the farmers, the city dwellers had little respect for mankind and nature, the very foundation of a farmer's livelihood. This was all reason enough for farmers to abstain from communicating with these strangers.

The consequences were grave in rural communities, including fewer opportunities for an education and a higher suicide rate, as its population rarely asked for counseling from the foreign world of urban psychology. The attitude of both sides stemmed from a lack of information about the other's true situation. Fortunately, both sides are beginning to develop channels of communication, bringing them closer together. And I am happy that I can be of help as a translator in this process.

The rural population was silent and remains silent for many good reasons. They have learned to observe closely and to recognize hidden interrelationships. To them, this knowledge is just part of the world, and the way to know it is by being part of the world yourself, observing, doing, and being—not by talking about it. They remain silent because they have learned not to be intrusive. They remain silent because they know exactly when it makes sense to disclose something to someone. They remain silent when someone is arrogant or patronizing, even if it is one of their children (one of many reasons why Number knowledge, the art of correct timing, and many other aspects of ancestral lore have been lost). They remain silent because the secrets of life and healing should only be placed in the hands of those who have shown the necessary sense of responsibility in their daily lives. It takes time to pass this test. And they have veiled their secret knowledge with small talk so that no one will discover the priceless knowledge they guard.

Building Bridges

Not too long ago, Johanna and I were watching a wonderful documentary about the Northern Bald Ibis, a unique species of bird that is being reintroduced to the wilderness of the Alps. One of key elements for the success of this project was that the birds had to learn to follow ultralight planes flown by their human caretakers south across the Alps. Sometimes the birds followed and sometimes they did not, leaving scientists at their wit's end. Sitting next to me, Johanna said, "Too bad they don't know that birds only fly on certain days and during certain lunar phases. Besides, they follow the energies of the Code. The date is always important."

Her comment got me thinking of the two worlds that I have learned to traverse over the decades. I feel that I have become a translator and facilitator between these worlds—the silent world of the Tyrolean mountain farmers, who developed thinking and observation skills, and the noisy world of the city dwellers, where knowledge only comes from outside sources, like books and the internet.

It also seems as if my path of upbringing, education, and professional life guided me specifically to this task of building bridges between worlds. I devoured hundreds of travel books in my childhood, and at sixteen, I rode a bicycle from Munich to London and back again, just to feel what traveling was really like. After high school, I traveled a great deal to meet the world's people, financed by my job of driving a taxi in Munich. I bought a travel typewriter to make translations of nonfiction books in my taxi at the cabstand, a newfound hobby that became part of my professional life later on.

However, I knew it was time to quit taxi driving when the customers started becoming unwelcome interruptions to my writing. I started writing nonfiction books with the intention of translating some of the reality that was out there for readers to understand. Slowly I came to realize that being an author is just that—translating what's out there.

For this reason, I am delighted to help build a bridge between the two worlds. It would be an irreplaceable loss if restraint on the one side and haughtiness and arrogance on the other made us forfeit this treasure trove of ancestral knowledge. Many of its elements are indispensable for a good future.

All in all, we hope that the Code shows you that you cannot judge a "book" by its cover. The silence, in other words, that can surround a person does not indicate anything about his or her knowledge and true worth—neither does loud advertising. Rather, as the old saying goes, "By their fruits, you shall know them." Some fruits just take longer to ripen than others, even though this can test the limits of one's patience.

Over the course of my own experience living day to day with the Code, it has transformed into an image of sublime beauty in my mind's eye. I marvel at the wonderful and ingenious Creator of this world who envisioned such a scenario. The Code leaves less leeway for coincidence in our daily lives, and we are granted a glance behind the scenes of the world theater. We learn about the loving, guiding powers that do everything to help us meet the challenges and tests we encounter.

The Code is one of the most precious tools our ancestors developed and passed on. It is valuable in so many situations, for people in all walks of life from all over the world, at every age without exception. It is a true treasure of possibilities and opportunities, beneficial for anyone who considers life an arena for maturation and ongoing personal development. Please accept this as a gift that will help you become and remain healthy and whole. Accept this out of love for yourself and love for life.

How to Use This Book

We ask you to read *The Code* in its entirety for your own benefit. Leave nothing out! Insights and connections are hidden in lines and paragraphs that you may think are worth skipping at first glance, and can yield a lot of important personal information for you. Once you have grasped all the colors of the rainbow, the full range of the Code's possibilities will open up to you, bringing your personal history and experience into a new, dynamic light.

In part 1, you'll be introduced to the key aspects of working with your Numbers, including the Birthday Wheel, your Cardinal Points, and your Signature. You will learn important terms and ideas that will help you better understand this book, and your own Code will start to take shape. In this section especially, as well as throughout the book, you may want to use a notebook to journal in or you can use the Code Journal pages at the back of the book in order to keep track of the information you discover about yourself and your loved ones.

In part 2, you'll learn about the building blocks of the Code through helpful details about the individual Numbers and the qualities they impart. You will discover suggestions for each Number: if you have them in your Code, if they are overdeveloped, if they are hiding, or if they are missing altogether.

Part 3 covers all of the possible Signatures that can be created from the Numbers. Here, you can read more about your individual Signature to gain insight into your nature and, of course, gain a better understanding of the Signatures of your friends, family, and professional associates as well.

Part 4 offers guidance on using the Code in your daily life. Here you will find tips on healing, working with children's Numbers, and geographic considerations, among other suggestions.

The Numbers found in the Code contain certain energies that are invoked by the use of color. Therefore, when presenting the Numbers in the text, we show them with their associated color. For example, the Numbers six and one, when used as part of the Code, are associated with the color blue and will be presented as ❻ and ❶.

Throughout the book, the Numbers of the Code are often discussed as linked pairs. A linked pair of Numbers consists of two different Numbers that have similar effects, such as the ❻ and ❶ shown above. There are five sets of linked Number pairs in the Code, and depending on what your specific Numbers are, it is possible to have one or both Numbers from a linked pair in your Code.

There can be a small amount of confusion that arises when discussing these linked pairs and so deserves a brief explanation. Since both Numbers in a linked pair impart many of the same effects in the Code, we often refer to linked pairs together because having either in your Code, say, the ❻ and/or ❶—or the ❼ and/or ❷—will give your Code many of the same general traits.

In section headings, we use the form "and/or" to present linked pairs (as on page 25—The People of the North: The Gift of the ❻ and/or ❶ in Your Birthdate), but we found this to be a bit wordy in the text. In order to strike a balance between absolute clarity of meaning and ease of reading, we have chosen to write about the linked pairs using only "or" or only "and" when appropriate. For example, when you have the ❻ *and* ❶ in your Code, you have them both. On the other hand, when the linked pairs are presented with just an "or," you may have either a ❻ or a ❶, both a ❻ and a ❶, or more than one occurrence of either or both Numbers in your Code.

For easy reference, we have also included a Numbers Chart on pages 262 and 263 that provides at-a-glance details of some of the book's key points. For example:

- Positive and negative aspects
- Professions and areas of proficiency
- Qualities
- Feminine and masculine energies

Let's get started!

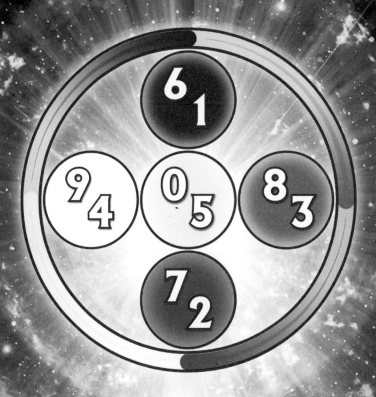

Part 1

Understanding the Code
of the Birthday Wheel

1

How to Find Your Personal Code

In this section, we will introduce the Birthday Wheel, show you an easy shorthand version of the wheel, demonstrate how to determine your personal Numbers from your specific date of birth, and then show you how your Numbers go into the Birthday Wheel.

Have no fear! Although it might seem complicated at first glance, the basics of finding your Code are easy. The first step is to draw a simple, shorthand version of the wheel called a compass. The second step is to determine which Numbers from your day of birth go into your Birthday Wheel. The third step is to place your Numbers in the wheel. And that is really all it takes to get started on your journey with the Code.

The Birthday Wheel

Simply put, your Code consists of the month, day, and year of your birth. Those Numbers are positioned within the Birthday Wheel, as shown on the next page and which you may recognize from the cover of this book. How your Numbers fit into the wheel and the specific qualities inherent in each of the individual Numbers of your Birthday determines the legacy of your own personal Code. Here is the Birthday Wheel:

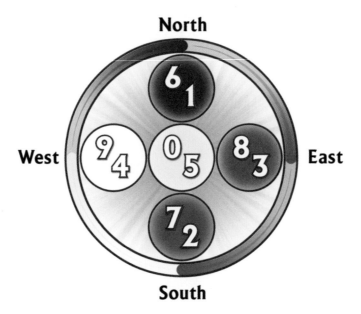

The basic structure of the Birthday Wheel always remains the same. Each direction of the compass—North, East, South, West, and Center—will always contain the same Numbers: ❻ and ❶ go into the North, ❽ and ❸ go into the East, ❼ and ❷ go into the South, ❾ and ❹ go into the West, and ⓿ and ❺ go into the center. Each direction also has its own color and holds its own special energy. What changes is how your individual Numbers fit into the Wheel to create your personal Code, and how you choose to use, or not use, the gifts of your Numbers and the Birthday Wheel.

In a moment, we will cover more details about the Birthday Wheel and how your individual Numbers are placed into the Wheel. First, we will show you a how to make a version of the wheel that can be created anywhere and makes finding your Code easy.

The Compass

In order to make the Code easier to understand, whether you are figuring out your own Numbers or the Numbers of a loved one, or you want to show someone at a dinner party or family get-together how the Numbers work, we have come up with a shorthand version of the Birthday Wheel, called the compass.

The compass can be quickly and easily drawn on whatever you have at hand, be it a napkin, Post-it note, piece of scrap paper, or journal. Plugging your Numbers into the compass is the best way to figure out your personal Code and how your Numbers work in the Birthday Wheel.

To make a compass, simply draw two lines that are roughly the same length, perpendicular to each other, and cross in the center. Then label the directions like a compass: North, East, South, West, and Center. That's it. Here is an example:

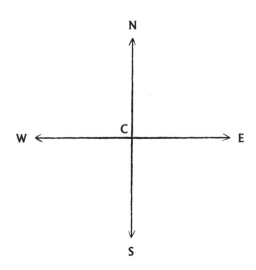

The Numbers of Your Code

Now that you know how to draw a compass, it's time to learn about the Numbers that make up each person's individual Code—month/day/year. You may want to read this whole section before filling out your first compass. In the next section, we will describe in detail the process of inputting the Numbers into the Birthday Wheel or shorthand compass.

Month Numbers

First, look at the Number or Numbers of your birth month, namely the Numbers 1 to 12, January to December. Were you were born in November? In this case, you will be adding a ❶ and a ❶ to your Birthday Wheel. Were you were born in October? Then you will be adding a ❶ and a ⓿ to your Wheel. You would not use a "placeholder" zero, however, if your birth month is a single digit number. For example, if you were born in June, you only have a ❻, not a ⓿ and ❻. Only those born in October have a ⓿ as a Number in their birth month.

Day Numbers

Second, look at the Number or Numbers of the day on which you were born, the day of the month ranging from 1 to 31. For example, if you were born on the 12th day of the month, then you will be entering the Numbers ❶ and ❷ into your Wheel. If you were born on the 5th, then you will be putting the Number ❺ into your Wheel. You would not use a "placeholder" zero if your birthdate is a single digit. Only those born on the 10th, 20th, or 30th of the month have a ⓿ in their birthdate.

Year Numbers

Third, find the Number or Numbers of your birth year. For example, if you were born in 1981 or 1959, the year Numbers are ❽ and ❶ or ❺ and ❾, respectively. For a person born in 2004, both the ⓿ and ❹ will be going in the personal birthday Code.

Year Numbers are significant in birthdates because they carry a bit more weight than the day and month Numbers, especially the Number in the ones column. For example, take two people with the same year Numbers: one person born in 1985 and the other in 1958. They both have the same Numbers in their Birthday Wheels, an ❽ and ❺, but the ❺ will mean more for the person born in 1985 than it will for the person born in 1958, who is more concerned about the ramifications of the ❽ in the birth year.

What about the century and millennial Numbers of your date of birth? Generally, the ❶ and ❾ of the twentieth century and the ❷ and ⓿ of the twenty-first century are not taken into account. We will say more on this subject in part 4, since these Numbers have a significant influence on world events. For the moment, however, we want to be sure that you know what forms your personal Code.

Your personal Code consists of a minimum of four to a maximum of six Numbers. For example:

- If you were born on July 5, 1966, then you have four Numbers: ❼, ⑤, ❻, and ❻.
- If you were born on September 12, 1947, then you have five Numbers: ❾, ❶, ❷, ❹, and ❼.
- If you were born on December 21, 1985, then you have six Numbers: ❶,❷,❷,❶,❽, and ⑤.

Placing Your Numbers in the Wheel

Draw a compass and label the North, East, South, West, and Center. You may find it helpful to write out the birthday in mm/dd/yy format somewhere on or near the compass. Remember to leave out the placeholder zeros that do not go into the Code.

Place the Numbers from your personal birthday Code into the compass as they correspond with the Numbers on the Birthday Wheel. Remember, the specific Numbers always go into the same location on the wheel: ❻ and ❶ go into the North, ❽ and ❸ go into the East, ❼ and ❷ go into the South, ❾ and ❹ go into the West, ⓪ and ⑤ go into the center. We find it helpful to draw a circle around each number as it is placed in the Wheel. Here are some examples:

Date of birth: July 4, 1955. The important Numbers of the Code here are ❼, ❹, ⑤ and ⑤. When you take a closer look at the first diagram on the next page, you will see where these Numbers belong: the ❼ is at the bottom in the South, the ❹ is entered on the left in the West, and the two ⑤s are entered in the Center position.

Date of birth: July 18, 1972. In this example, you would add ❼, ❶, ❽, ❼, ❷ to the Wheel in accordance with their corresponding directions (see the second diagram on the next page).

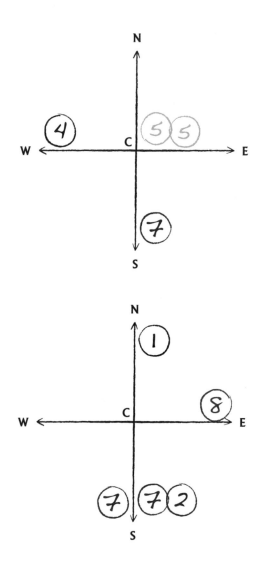

The Cardinal Points

Each pair of Numbers on the Birthday Wheel has been assigned a direction, known as a Cardinal Point. Your Cardinal Points are the directions in which your Numbers are located. For example, if your birthday is 6/1/50, you occupy the Cardinal Points North and Center. You may also see the term "Station" used to describe a Cardinal Point. The term Station is helpful when talking about the motion of the wheel. Energy in the wheel always moves in a clockwise direction. Therefore, when you read that the South is being energized by the previous Station of the Wheel, we are referring to the East.

The following diagram will help you find your Cardinal Points. Make note of them in your Code Journal if you have decided to keep one.

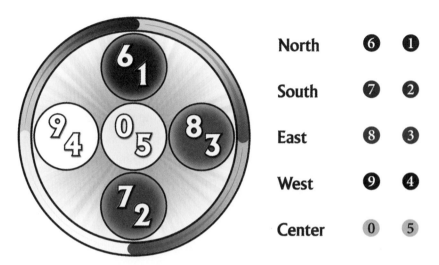

Geographic locations also hold the energy of the Number Wheel, the reason why Texans and New Yorkers are so different from each other. Even within the structure of an individual state, the meaning of the pairs is so profound that the people of the South are different from those of the East or the West. We discuss this significance in greater detail in part 4.

You will gradually grow into this knowledge as you get more experienced, and your self-confidence will grow. You will be able to understand the enormous upheaval caused by the reunification of West and East Germany or the split of the North from the South in the American Civil War. In part 3, we briefly address what happens when, for example, a South becomes a North virtually overnight (see page 231).

Number Colors

Next, find your Number Color. Each individual Number in your birthdate has a corresponding color that carries with it the energy of that specific Number and its location on the Number Wheel. When you look at the

Wheel, shown throughout the book or on the cover, you will be able to see the connection:

- ◆ Blue and black for ❻ and ❶
- ◆ Green for ❽ and ❸
- ◆ Red for ❼ and ❷
- ◆ White for ❾ and ❹
- ◆ Yellow for ⓪ and ⑤

It is very important to know the corresponding colors for the Numbers, as we will demonstrate in the following chapters. For example, wearing certain colors can balance the influence of the Numbers in yourself or in people with whom you are in contact frequently.

The Signatures

Your Signature comes from your personal Number Code and is made up of the Cardinal Points in which your Numbers are located (North, East, South, West, and Center). Let's say you were born on September 5, 1961, then your personal Numbers are in the North, West, and Center of the compass. When plotting out the Numbers, a certain symbolic picture emerges on the Birthday Wheel. In this case, it is the formation of the North, West, and Center. We refer to this formation as a Signature.

There are thirty-one Number combinations possible and, therefore, thirty-one individual Signatures. Find your Signature—your combination of Cardinal Points—and note it in your Code Journal at the back of the book if you wish. In part 3, you will learn what your Signature reveals about you and how you can use it to your advantage.

Weighing the Units

The sum of the Units in each of your Cardinal Points is merely the sum of its Numbers. For example, if someone was born on October 9, 1959, the West shows the Number ❾ twice. Therefore, this person has eighteen Units of the energy that dominate the West of the Wheel.

In your Code Journal, add up the number of Units in each Cardinal Point of your Wheel. The ⓪ counts for ten Units. Make note of any Cardinal Point that has more than ten Units. If your date of birth shows more than ten Units at any of the Cardinal Points, it could possibly lead to extreme overdevelopment. You will learn in the following pages what effect such an overload might have.

To go back to our example, if you have the Number ❾ once in your personal Code, it indicates in most cases that you have good business sense. If the ❾ appears twice, it might border on the extreme and turn into selfishness, stinginess, and willfulness. The "savvy business sense" may change to "compulsive clinging" or "repulsive avarice." In this instance, the ⓪ and ⑤ in the birthdate are a good counterbalance to the weightiness of the West since they add up to fifteen Units in the Center.

Masculine and Feminine

There is another important difference in the Numbers. The higher Numbers—❻, ❼, ❽, ❾, and ⓪—represent feminine energy. They are overall tougher, more tenacious, and more enduring. They lack, however, the spontaneity of the lower masculine Numbers—❶, ❷, ❸, ❹, and ⑤. The masculine Numbers at each Station have an immediate and resounding effect, but they are not long-lasting.

One example of this difference can be seen in people whose date of birth shows only the Numbers ❶ through ⑤. In general, you would meet a more fast-moving character, less burdened by indecisiveness but more prone to impatience and recklessness, even in everyday dealings. The other extreme—birthdays with only the Numbers ❻ through ⓪—are more patient and thoughtful to the point of hesitation, even in situations requiring quick reflexes. These differences will become apparent as you gather experience using the Code over time.

The Center of Gravity

The individual distribution of Numbers within a Signature displays the unique arrangement of the prevalent energies, existing talents, and inherent abilities of that person. Therefore, it is important to closely examine the Numbers that make up each Signature. Where is the "Center of Gravity"? As an example, compare the birthdates May 1, 1966, and May 10, 1955. Both have an identical Signature, with the qualities of the North and the Center providing the general direction. However, in each case a different character will emerge based on the treasure chest of energies and assets available to it. The former birthdate gravitates more to the North, whereas the latter is "colored" by the Center, which has its own little treasure trove of different elements. This will be covered in much greater detail in parts 2 and 3.

In part 2, we will also bring to life the Numbers of your birthdate. Be patient, however, while we take the next chapter to further illuminate important aspects of the Birthday Wheel, namely its inner movement and its dynamics. We will also reveal what this could and should mean to you.

At this point, you should be familiar with your Numbers, Cardinal Points, Colors, and Signature. You should also be aware of the Units in each of your Cardinal Points and where your Center of Gravity is located. These are the basic tools for harnessing the power of your personal Code. Keep this information easily accessible in your notebook or Code Journal, as it will be helpful to you throughout the book.

2

The Spiral Journey of
the Birthday Wheel

What you are about to read may seem a bit confusing at first, but do not worry. You are already familiar with a similar effect. When you first read the somewhat mysterious instructions for your new computer, a new kitchen appliance, or a new cell phone, for example, it takes a few days of trial and error to understand them. Eventually, however, the various functions and steps become second nature. If you practice with the Birthday Wheel for a while and then reread the following chapter, you will find that everything feels familiar and natural. So take heart!

The Wheel in Motion

Take a look at the Birthday Wheel on the front cover of this book. The Numbers of the Wheel are arranged in a circle that moves clockwise from Station to Station. This is the natural direction of all movement within the Birthday Wheel. It starts in the North, rotates to the East, South, and West, and then back up to North, with Center in constant participation like the hub of a wheel.

Food is likewise energized by this clockwise motion, whether you are stirring your tea or coffee or using your wooden spoon to mix ingredients. As strange as this may sound now, all will become clearer in the following pages and over time as you experience and observe the Code in your surroundings. The most detailed description of a lemon's tartness does not prepare you for actually tasting it.

Since the Wheel reflects the workings of nature, living by the Birthday Wheel and its Stations leads to success for everything and everyone. It begins at the end of the old and the seed of the new idea (North), moves to the enthusiasm and deep joy in the developmental stage (East), continues on to the lively and enthusiastic process of presentation (South), advances into the smart, successful, safe, and flawlessly functioning logistical phase (West), and finally steps into the limelight (North). From there, we experience further fine-tuning and upward movement as the process continues around the Wheel once again.

Balancing the Wheel

There is also another reason for the spiral nature of the Wheel. It is a person's life task to fill the empty Stations and Cardinal Points in his or her personal Code. Essentially, there are two ways to do this: align with partners whose dates of birth contain the Numbers we lack in our own Signatures or familiarize ourselves with the missing Numbers' special energies and abilities.

Filling these voids is, above all else, a matter of personal intuition, but it can be formulated as follows: First, it is important to understand the significance of the missing Numbers and the special powers and abilities associated with them. The traits of these Numbers should not be acquired in order to become just like the people who have them in their dates of birth. Rather, they should be acquired in order to create harmony in its widest sense—in order to understand people better and to feel comfortable in your own skin. A master chef who creates the most heavenly dishes will never feel completely at ease inwardly if he or she does not develop a basic feeling of what makes a master waiter. The president of a great country will never be his people's first servant and rule wisely if he hasn't tasted the life of a servant; he must feel true empathy for all of his country's citizens.

Secondly (and this is where the spiral movement comes into play), this means that you should pass your own Numbers and their inherent abilities (namely, your special knowledge and talents) to the empty Stations in your Signature. This should be done clockwise and can be accomplished best by teaching your own knowledge and wisdom to people with Stations missing from your Signature. This process will become clearer later on.

Parents and early childhood professionals observe every day the inherent dedication in children to fill the voids in their personal Signatures. Children intuitively experiment with all sorts of activities even though they did not enter the world with the related abilities.

Unfortunately, many children encounter discouragement at an early age, such as when people say to them, "That can't be real!" or "How much longer are you going to take?" As a result, many children will not tackle life's adventures again until they reach adulthood. However, it is never too late to become whole and healthy.

As we mentioned in the last chapter, Number Colors are a useful way of filling your voids. For example, you should get to know the Numbers and corresponding colors of everyone with whom you have had close contact with over an extended period of time (relatives, friends, colleagues, students, and so on). Otherwise, you could feel strangely drained and nervous in their presence at times. This happens frequently when both sides have a void in the same Cardinal Point (North, East, South, West, or Center) and its corresponding color. You can, however, apply your knowledge of the connection between the Numbers of the Birthday Wheel and their colors in order to successfully counteract the loss of energy. For example, you could wear clothes with colors that are missing from your Signature.

On the other hand, if the person you are with has Numbers that contain several Units of a Number and color that your date of birth is missing (for example, two **6**s where you have no North Station), then this person's mere presence can be beneficial to you. This person also benefits because your presence helps balance his or her overload of blue/black. The presence of a person can make us ill or healthy, as you may know from experience.

◆ ◆ A Story from Johanna ◆ ◆

For many years, after moving from the Austrian Alps to the big city of Munich, I naturally paid attention to the colors in my surroundings. When I visited friends, I would often wonder why there was very little of a certain color in their immediate surroundings.

For example, in one house, the color red was virtually nonexistent, even though the hosts definitely lacked energy. It took me a while to realize that they were not familiar with such healing methods. If anything, they might have called these methods pure superstition. Years later, when these same people needed help with various illnesses, they came back to me for advice. I recommended that they see a holistic healer and suggested color and Number work as additional support. It worked well for them and in many cases later, with others who would call themselves "nonbelievers." I didn't explain or justify my recommendations, but simply let the results speak for themselves.

The Wheel in Practice

The Wheel is ancient knowledge that has been used for centuries. Farmers and workers have known its powers and have implemented it in their livelihoods in order to see their ideas come to fruition. Let's see the Wheel in motion with the help of a real-world example. We'll use the development of an idea for a product and its implementation.

Inception: "I have an idea!"

The creative process can begin anywhere and is not tied to a particular Station; this door is open to everyone. Let's say your date of birth contains the North (**6** or **1**) and the Center (**0** or **5**) (and, therefore, has the Signature North–Center), and you have a terrific idea for a new board game. In order to transform this idea into a successfully realized task using the Code, we must set the Wheel in motion. What follows first is the transfer of your idea to the East, where all ideas must take their first steps. What does that mean? Let us explain.

Development: "It is a good idea!"

After an idea for a product begins somewhere in the universe, the first Station on its path to realization is the East; that is, it becomes affiliated with a person whose date of birth contains the East or with a company whose specialty is to pick up new ideas, develop, and implement them. Such companies are always "companies of the East" because it is highly likely that employees with an ❽ or ❸ play important roles there. Their Wheels and lives are meant to accompany and monitor the realization of ideas during their initial stages. They are the ones who are able to create the prototype of your idea.

Presentation: "It is a good thing. Everybody look!"

In the next step, the East passes the prototype on to the South (❼ or ❷). If the first company also has the characteristics of the South integrated, it will take the next step itself, or another company with Numbers in the South will take over. At this point, the next step is to make a convincing presentation of the product on a small scale—at a trade fair, for example, where the product can be noticed by a larger audience. One of the most beautiful things in the creative process is a successful presentation that stirs up enthusiasm for the product (a typical feat of the people of the South). Your personal task here in the South is to monitor and accompany your product to ensure that your philosophy has been preserved in the process and is seen through to its ultimate completion and release.

Realization: "See how feasible it is!"

The South has now opened the way to pass your brainchild, the terrific board game, to the West (❾ or ❹). The West can at times be a spoilsport and put a damper on your enthusiasm, but that is often necessary. The West is the home of the serious development of your initial thought into a mature idea or product. Here you will find the balance between what is ideal and what is feasible, between the perfection of what you dream about and its practical realization. This includes smart calculations and price strategy, advertising and publicity, target group selection, adept marketing, logistics and distribution—everything necessary to bring a good product to the public that is representative of the inherent qualities of the people of the West. Your task is to monitor and supervise this process. You might also want to hire a good tax adviser who will keep a close eye on sound finances.

Maturation: "You can have it now!"

This final step completes the journey around the Birthday Wheel to the North, where the game is handed over to the customer. The North, therefore, is not only the birthplace of the idea but also the completion of its maturation and its readiness to be handed over to the world. Let's say you have the North (❻ or ❶) in your Birthday Wheel, including its wealth of ideas and the savvy for launching fully formulated ideas to the public. As a result, you can now take a number of matters into your own hands.

This example of developing the board game shows that you do not have to do everything yourself when it comes to the empty Stations of your Code. You should merely keep the ball rolling by understanding the inherent abilities that lie in Stations other than your own, assisting when possible and overseeing the work. Our example can be applied to all situations and Signatures. By substituting "special knowledge" (or "music," "healing," "invention," and others) for "board game," you will come much closer to understanding the heart of the Code.

Let's assume that in your Code all Cardinal Points are present except for the West, like in March 26, 1951. In this case, you can successfully guide the product maturation process, with the exception of sound financial planning, accounting, advertising, and the application of commercial standards. Those belong in the hands of people with an occupied West in their Wheel. All that is required is that you be intelligent about contracts, and monitor the logistics and activities of the West.

Lift Yourself Up with Each Rotation

Let's summarize what happens within the circular movement of the Wheel. Even though a wheel's circumference has no end, the Birthday Wheel's primary inner energy starts its invisible rotational in the North with the ❻ and ❶. The North simultaneously represents both the end and the high point of development as well as the start of a new cycle. It is like the quiet before a new beginning or the collecting energy for a new circumstance, like winter before spring. The beginnings of a new development are already present but not yet readily noticeable.

In the East, however, where the ❽ and ❸ are present, the new development is already fully at work and moving along. Spring is in full bloom.

The South, which contains the ❼ and ❷, represents the power of summer, the full enjoyment of energies—vitality. In this stage, preparations and initial guidance are now finished. All things hidden are now expressed, formed, and shaped.

The West, with the ❾ and ❹, fortifies the success, presents it, and makes it useful for posterity. Then the North completes the circular movement by bringing what has matured out into the open, making it available to everyone. It adds a special something that will plant the seed for the next round, which begins again in the North with the ❻ and ❶.

The Numbers in the Center (⓪ and ⑤) carry something from each Station; you can go anywhere from the Center. The Center can be used as a wild card in order to bring empty Stations to life. Life has more than one cycle.

The Wheel does not circle with endless repetitions. Instead, it moves to the beginning of a qualitatively higher developmental plane, a spiral that becomes stronger and stronger when the energy is moving well.

You lift yourself up with each completed rotational cycle. As an idea is realized, knowledge is transferred, and good things are manifested with each completed rotation of the Wheel. As seen from above, the Wheel is a two-dimensional, colored circle, but when seen from all sides, the Wheel becomes a colorful, three-dimensional spiral winding toward heaven!

As time passes, you might want to occasionally reflect upon this beautiful shape as your understanding of its interrelations grow. You may even reach the point where you do not think of things as "jumping" from Station to Station and instead perceive them as having an uninterrupted flow.

Our language knows terms like baby, toddler, child, teenager, and adult. But on your eighteenth birthday, were you really much smarter and more grown up than you were the day before? Everything in life flows and intertwines, much of it seamlessly. This is also true for the Birthday Wheel. Extreme developments and inner stagnation occur when we do not leave enough room for the natural flow of life. The Native Americans have a wonderful allegory for this: "Only a bubbling stream that freely gives its water away will remain fresh and clear. Standing water becomes a foul-smelling swamp."

From the very beginning, everyone is destined to follow a calling. This also becomes apparent from the Wheel's composition. If we actualize this calling, success will come—and with it the obligation to pass it on materially, intellectually, and emotionally. Success kept to oneself never means true success and happiness, and it frequently burns out quickly. Share your treasure with others so that everyone will benefit!

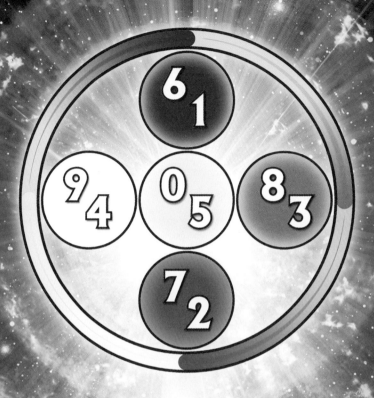

Part 2

The Building Blocks
of the Code

Introduction to the Building Blocks

Each Number in your date of birth represents a gift that was placed in your treasure chest. This unique cache of Numbers was given to you to help you to successfully complete certain tasks that you encounter in your life.

Each individual Number in the Code essentially stands for two things: a special task that needs to be completed and the existence of all of the tools required to complete this task successfully. We find out where the journey will lead and are then given the necessary money for the fare. The challenge consists of recognizing our individual path and traversing various territories until we reach our goal. Even though it sometimes may not appear that we have the freedom to choose whether to get on the train or allow ourselves to be sidetracked, we do. We are the conductors of our life's path.

Throughout each chapter, you will find quotes that we refer to as "medicine for the soul." The quotes, tailored to the particular Station, will help you fully understand the gift of the Numbers.

Please read all of the chapters in this section. If your date of birth does not contain the Numbers of a particular Station, you will still find information on how to work with those missing Numbers. The chapters address many thoughts and connections that are relevant to all Numbers.

3

The North (❻ and ❶)

Charisma, Vision, and Determination

The People of the North: The Gift of the ❻ and/or ❶ in Your Birthdate

These Numbers are like stepping stones on the path into the public eye. They give you inner strength and provide the kind of vibrations that will allow you to be heard everywhere. These Numbers lend charisma and vibrancy; the bearers of these Numbers do not work in silence. They openly display all of their acquired talents and abilities, their knowledge and experiences, and pass them on to the general public, not just to their own children. This holds true even if you are one of those people who is overcome by stage fright at the mere thought of giving a speech in front of a large group of people. When people with the North in their date of birth experience fear and shyness, it is generally the result of childhood experiences, psychological injuries, and underdeveloped self-confidence.

As long as the ❻ or the ❶ are present, you will always find the power and charisma necessary for a courageous and successful public appearance, even if those powers are hidden behind a fog of timidity. People will listen to you. You have the necessary tools and strength. The ❻ and ❶ provide the talent to build bridges among people.

The ❻ and ❶ provide willpower, assertiveness, and endurance. There are so many causes in this world that are still unresolved and require loving dedication of these Numbers. For example, it is only in answering questions about the true cause of terrorism that a permanent solution can be found. The ❻ and ❶ impart visionary qualities to their bearers so that their hearts and intellect can devote themselves to solving these questions about the future.

Furthermore, people of the North persevere when striving for goals. They do not immediately give up, even when faced with sizable obstacles. Indeed, they often do not perceive obstacles as anything other than a part of life's natural rhythm, much like having aching muscles after strenuous exercise. This attitude helps them reach goals more easily than those without a ❻ or ❶ in their Code.

Long after others say, "This won't work," people of the North still dare to pursue avenues for resolution with vigorous and purposeful determination. They might even be ahead of their times. And then, a hundred years later, the outstanding quality and genius of their work become apparent, when the world is on the same wavelength and the necessary vibrations are present. This forward thinking is also one of the roots of unhappiness for people of the North, as being ahead of one's time can be a lonely road.

People of the North rarely find happiness in regimented civil service jobs. Instead, they find their heart's calling as pioneers, reformers, lawyers, philosophers, writers, politicians, and diplomats. They do well as teachers (because they will have a receptive audience and will teach wisely), as judges (because they are able to look beyond the obvious to see things clearly and with depth), or as researchers (especially with a ❾ or ❹ in their date of birth, which fosters the necessary self-discipline). Actors can also be found in the palette of professions of the North. Those who enter the world's stage without the presence of the ❻ or ❶ in their date of birth generally have a rough road to success. Of course, this does not mean that their road to success is closed. The passion of the ❼ and ❷ also opens doors to the world.

The inquisitive mind makes its home everywhere and is a part of every person's soul, whether it is actively expressed or not. In the North, however, in order to be happy, it is essential that the inquisitive mind be actively engaged. Not only that, but the ❻ and ❶ are not satisfied with superficial signs of progress and are able to see through the pseudo-progress of trends. They are not easily caught up in passing fads or in the "latest" scientific findings. They are so passionate about the truth that they are not fooled by pretense, at least not in the long run.

For these reasons, the ❻ and ❶ are assigned the qualities of water. Water flows everywhere, much like the ❻ and ❶, and these Numbers represent the same curious, searching spirit that will not rest until it has found answers. The energy of the ❻ and ❶ also corresponds to the coolness of a bubbling stream's water and works efficiently. Its energy reaches everyone on the planet, even in the remotest of corners.

The ❻ and ❶ are at home in every aspect of public relations work, whether in the world of the media or in the humanities. The pioneering spirit is so much at home in the North that people of the North can become bored and depressed. This happens when they are forced to perform routine tasks day in and day out that do not offer at least partial success, or in situations where everyone around them is doing the same thing. In the long run, living strictly for hearth and home will not bring happiness to the person of the North, unless by doing so he or she contributes to someone else's success. Therefore, the ❻ and ❶ tend to play a leading role, sometimes very much under the radar. They like to consider all other Numbers to be helpers along their way.

Perhaps you are now wondering if the ❻ and ❶ each generate the same energy; there is very little observable difference between them. However, the ❶ might represent knowledge and communication to a somewhat greater degree; the ❶ is more inquisitive. And while the ❻ is more easily satisfied and content with its accomplishments, its thirst for knowledge never subsides.

You may have guessed that, in the current state of the world, it is not easy for the ❻ and ❶ to actualize their curiosity and sense of adventure when every billboard and television advertisement spews an insidious, subliminal invitation to lead a comfortable life as a consumer. In the long term, it will take much willpower, self-love, and self-discipline to resist these attempts to undermine the power of the North.

There are few schools and companies that teach the art of "thinking things through to their logical conclusion." Sadly, the development of free will and self-confidence are not encouraged enough. If they were, more people would be able to resist the temptation to succumb without struggle to stagnation and self-numbing. Consequently, a person of the North might find the most wonderful, ideally suited partner for an exciting, fulfilling life journey of mutual development but then part ways with a heavy (or even light) heart because this partner refuses to grow up, having been bribed into the "normal" lifestyle of unreflective consumerism. Of course, there will always be natural-born "little housewives" or "substitute daddies" to happily fill in as partners for this eternal child, but this is unlikely to bring true happiness.

The North is happy only when it is actually moving. The pretense of movement or sitting at a standstill will rob it of its vitality.

Fortunately, the Birthday Wheel is never still, as each Station brings its own dimension of movement. In the North, the ❻ and the ❶ contribute the intense quiet before a new start. This is an immensely fertile phase that provides the seed for many life journeys. At the same time, this is also the completion of the circle, having gone from the conception of an idea to its realization. And this in turn makes room for new ideas.

Children of the North

Children and teens whose date of birth contains the ❻ or the ❶ always have to experience something new, and their curiosity should be encouraged and supported. If their parents have become resigned and devote themselves to the superficial things in life, like a muted evening in front of the television with a beer, then the children of the North can become a chronic nuisance. The reason for this is simply a lack of parental understanding; the parents have blocked the connection to their children. And this behavior often goes hand in hand with parents cutting themselves off from other people.

When children of the North are not able to express their talents, they unconsciously use various methods to fight against their impairment. For these oppressed children, acquiescence and "becoming just like Mom or Dad" is the very last thing they want, and they will actively look for ways out of the situation.

A rarely recognized, deeper reason for the problems of some of the children of the North stems from frequently being called "too slow" by parents, siblings, and teachers, but nothing could be further from the truth. These children are simply engrossed with thoroughness and dedication in their endeavors, and have minds that quickly travel into realms beyond the imagination of their critics at home and in school. Children of the North learn more in ten minutes of quiet musing than others learn in three hours of serious study.

In reality, these children want nothing more than to know things in detail. They rarely do something only because others are doing it; they are not followers. Headstrong, they want special treatment and scrutinize everything.

But please look closely. Their intense questioning is not to be confused with the endless chatter of ill-mannered children. Ill manners are rooted in parental weakness. But woe if the children of the North also have a strong West, the ❾ or ❹, in their date of birth. If this is the case, they can get their way even when it is not appropriate, and sometimes with brutal stubbornness.

All in all, children who have the ❻ or ❶ in their date of birth are headed in the right direction. They merely need gentle guidance and much understanding as they realize that they will still be successful in life even if they take a different path from their parents.

Shadows on the North: The Promise Not Yet Fulfilled

In our conversations with interested readers and people who attend our talks, we often get the same question: "Why is it that after we learn the Code and read the Numbers for ourselves or someone close to us, we are still convinced that we are facing a total opposite of what it says?"

Why is it that we do not recognize the energy of the Stations of the Birthday Wheel in ourselves? For example, how is it possible that the bearer of the ❻ or ❶ can arrange his or her business and personal life in such a way that everything always remains the same?

Or what if we feel and recognize our Number energy but don't give it room to enter our lives so that we can become truly happy ourselves (like the bearer of the ❻ or ❶ above, who is afraid of all changes but secretly yearns for new experiences)?

By now, you know that each Number of your birthdate points to a treasure trove of talents and abilities, or for some, a tendency toward exaggeration or fanaticism. In extreme cases, it can happen that these treasures will never be unearthed. Imagine that you have the talent to be a journalist or writer (when the ❻ or ❶ are present in your date of birth), but you were born into a family with strong mathematical and scientific leanings. Or maybe you were born into a family of physicians who have groomed you to follow in the footsteps of your father to eventually take over his practice.

In such situations, it could easily happen that the abilities and talents received from your Numbers never surface. You might only experience a strange, melancholy feeling (or similar movement of your soul) when reading a good book, or you may feel a vague longing that comes when you are leaning against the guardrail of a ship, watching the seagulls. There are many tradespeople who would have found their true fulfillment as writers or teachers, just as there are many physicians who are longing to sow a field or build a massive piece of furniture out of wood for all to enjoy.

When you recognize these interrelationships and are aware that you are living much differently than your Numbers indicate, it does not automatically mean that you are doomed to never be truly happy (because you sidestepped your true calling in life).

First, it is never too late to develop the natural gifts conveyed through your Numbers. The gift of the ❻ and ❶ is never wasted, nor is it ever drained to the last drop. It might even happen that you will write highly interesting articles or an exciting novel about this profession that does not really suit you.

Or you might say, "I dig and dig, but I do not recognize myself in the description, even though I have the North in my date of birth." Remember, the description of the remaining Numbers is yet to come. It may be that your purpose in life is different from what you have read so far.

As long as you can read these lines, you can make a fresh start. Never become discouraged. Instead, bring the hidden to light—it really does exist! Calmly ask yourself what it is that you truly want, and give yourself time for the answer. You might feel frustrated because you have forgotten how to ask this question, causing your true wishes to retreat to your subconscious. Independent of your achievements, ask yourself, "Which of these plans can I implement?"

The North is assigned the colors blue and black. For example, blue clothing could help you when you do not feel any part of the ❻ or ❶ in your life. Blue or black serves as a door-opener, as homeopathic medicine, as an invitation to the Cosmos to send you what is needed for your very own. When you recognize yourself in the description of the Numbers and feel the energy of the Numbers, working with the assigned color is not necessarily required, but it can be helpful.

When dealing with problems, it is important to ask, "How did I allow myself to get into this situation? What went wrong?" After all, nothing happens without reason. Maybe you have a third failed marriage. Perhaps you experience the same problems over and over with your children, your clients, or your boss. You may be making multiple moves between homes but always have the same difficulties with the neighbors. None of this is just chance or happenstance; we reap what we sow. Problems mean that we did not learn and internalize a certain lesson.

◆ ◆ ◆ ◆ ◆

No matter what your Numbers, you are sure to find the following exercise helpful:

Draw the Birthday Wheel and add your personal Numbers. Determine which Stations are empty. Use this book to see what each Cardinal Point stands for and what the missing Stations represent. Look at what you have in your life now and what you could have had instead. What is missing?

Then quietly meditate on the following questions:

What am I today?
What could I be?

There are sons and daughters for whom nothing is more important than taking over the family business. And then there are children who shudder at the mere idea of following in Dad's or Mom's footsteps. When one of these views is deeply ingrained, it does not matter what your Numbers are. When the urge to go out into the world is overpowering, or the main wish is to stay close to home, the extreme has already gotten the upper hand, rendering one's Numbers irrelevant. However, if you can tell by the Numbers that going out into the world is your child's birthright and duty, then you should not nag your child to take over the carpentry business, the farm, or the medical practice.

In the realm of the Code, nothing is cast in stone. There are no rules to be memorized. In the realm of Nature, countless natural causal relationships elude the cut-and-dried, scientific ways of thinking. The modern "computer method" frequently means judging, categorizing, establishing, labeling, and immobilizing. But nature does not work that way. That is one of its most beautiful attributes.

If you do not live out your Numbers but are happy nonetheless, then there is no reason to struggle to develop new abilities and hobbies. However, your natural talents should be set free when their lack of expression makes you unhappy or when you are saddened by a deep longing.

When the North Needs Taming: Development into the Extreme

The forward-looking, optimistic energy of the North, like every Number of the Wheel, runs the risk of becoming bloated when pushed to exaggeration or to the extreme. This frequently happens when the special powers of the North are suppressed. Feeling stifled or castrated, as it were, could lead to despair and depression. An increased need for rest or the feeling of overwhelming boredom are often merely the symptoms of stagnation and resignation. Thinking, "By the time they understand how important this is, I will probably be ready to retire," is typical of a person of the North who encounters limiting boundaries.

When the energy of the North is unusually strong (this is the case when the ❻ or the ❶ appears twice or even three times in someone's birth-date), it can result in manic-depressive tendencies, where you are on top of the world one minute and severely depressed the next. In this case, the challenge and learning experience involves the practice of patience as a counterbalance to your inborn impatience with daily drudgery.

It is not always easy to be around a person of the North. When he or she is forced to warn and prod others to take care of daily chores efficiently, this person can become quite cranky. For a person of the North, one true test of patience arises from people who escape their life's tasks by losing themselves in pets, video games, or other activities instead of engaging in the world. A bearer of the North would most likely turn away from such a person because it would be clear that his or her diversions are more impor-tant than fulfilling a life task.

A hunger for power can also be found in the North; with great ability and knowledge comes great temptation. A person of the North could, for example, begin to consider his or her assumed or actual level of knowledge as a sign of rank. Feeling superior is one of the most destructive poisons of the soul. It is truly a devilish matter. And the temptation is especially great when the ❾ or ❹ are also present in the date of birth, as this will increase narcissistic tendencies.

Sometimes, people of the North can also come across as being pushy and extremist, and because of their natural efficiency, they do not adjust gladly to the slower pace of others. When the genius of the people of the North does not find the ideal environment, these people can feel easily insulted, bored, or irritable. At times, they can give the appearance of being condescending or indifferent because they feel it is beneath them to deal with everyday routines or with anything they consider primitive. They can also become anxious when they, being highly sensitive people, hurt others. The pain caused by their forceful ways makes them afraid of the consequences.

Those whose North has more than ten Units should avoid wearing the colors blue and black above the waist and should be careful on days that contain the Numbers ❻ or ❶. The ❻ and ❶ belong to the night, when we are more receptive to new things. For this reason, the large amount of radiation that engulfs us these days (wireless internet, Bluetooth devices, cordless phones, cell phones and their towers) are especially damaging for the ❻ and ❶. People of the North would do well to avoid these radiation hotspots and the "blessings" brought on by our modern society, as much as possible.

The color of the opposite Station can be helpful in neutralizing and healing an extreme overdevelopment. In the case of the North, it would be the color of the South—red. It can be quite helpful to surround yourself with people whose birthdate contains the South (❼ or ❷), especially when you have neither the ❼ nor ❷ in your birthdate.

A strong sign of genuine development and maturation in your life, as in the life of every person, is the impulse to pass your treasures (knowledge, material goods, time, love, and so on) to other people—in particular, those who have Stations that you are lacking. In the case of the North, it would be the East, to people who have the ❽ or ❸ in their date of birth. This transfer has a healing effect.

When the North Is Missing: The Birthdate without the ❻ and/or ❶

A special adventure in the quest to learn the personal Code of your Birthday Wheel is to comprehend and incorporate your missing Stations and Numbers. And it is sufficient to fully understand the significance of the missing components without actualizing what is missing by choosing a profession that is tailored to the empty Station. Making a conscious effort to understand what is missing and fill the voids is enough. For example, if your North is empty, you can complete your personal Code by making an effort to form, voice, and stand by your own opinion.

The ❻ and ❶ deliver the innate insight that we must broaden our knowledge and that there is always more to learn. For those who do not have the North in their date of birth, they might feel they know enough already. This is demonstrated when a graduate thinks that he already has done everything needed to take on a job and live up to its expectations.

Those who do not make an effort to understand the significance of their missing Stations may sense deep down that an important aspect of their existence lies in the shadows. To not make this effort is to deny the core of our existence—the ability to be receptive, to grow, and to mature. Those who remain stuck in their judgments and prejudices wither away emotionally long before they die physically. In addition, he or she becomes a ready instrument for negative powers that require rigid thinking to fuel their own fires. Tyranny, arbitrariness, and mental slavery only have a chance when their "sheep" enjoy being dependent.

When Numbers are missing, it is not important to tame and incorporate their inherent energies. However, it is crucial to understand them and to learn how to deal with them. Generally, without the ❶, it is more difficult to develop unfaltering willpower. Often, as a substitute, we develop a tendency to be stubborn and unreasonable. Without the ❻ in our date of birth, it takes us somewhat longer to understand the need for necessary compromises.

When dealing with a child with a missing North, we might find ourselves repeating the same thing a thousand times. The child may even fake understanding, but then nothing happens. When observing adults with this same tendency, you may find that they are thinking of other things while talking. They are not aware of it themselves and do not consider this a weakness; they actually consider it a positive trait since they are mentally a few steps ahead. In reality, they overestimate themselves. Without concentrating on the present, they often miss important information. Their apparent progressiveness and speed in the long term transform into regression. By pushing ahead prematurely, one overlooks the important flow of information around them—one step forward, two steps back.

When the North is missing, it might take longer for us to notice that we need to change our behavior or life philosophy. Without the North, we can mistakenly look for a guilty party and blame external influences as the source for our difficulty. People with an empty North can be true artists when it comes to ignoring the cause. This happens especially when the true reasons are hidden under external worries and problems. A mere glance in the mirror would show where the solution is to be found, but people without the North in their Wheel are not natural "detectives of their own soul."

The Numbers of the North provide the ability to be objective—to step away from oneself to take a cool, honest look at oneself and others. Accordingly, the lack of the ❻ and ❶ sometimes translates into a lack of objectivity, the severity of which depends on how well we managed to get through childhood with this deficiency. The more successfully we get through childhood, the less we will regard the absence of ❻ and ❶'s clear vision and objectivity as a shortcoming, or challenge ourselves to fill this void in our character. Dealing with people who shirk personal responsibility can be draining because, as the saying goes, "It's like talking to a wall." Attempts at resolution tend to be in vain, especially in the long term.

The ❻ and ❶ confer a fine, penetrating perception. Many day-to-day problems, economic difficulties, and political issues cannot be solved without such perception and capacity for insight. Those who do not consider themselves part of the problem are unlikely to be part of the solution. If someone is stuck in a traffic jam and complains bitterly about it, he should keep in mind that he, too, is sitting in a car; he is the traffic jam. It is only this first step toward the truth that will lead to the strength and inspiration for true improvement.

People without the ❻ or ❶ can be loveable and valuable, go through life without offending anyone, and do great work for themselves and others. However, they can also frustrate people who have the North in their birthdate by denying the need for drastic changes in certain situations. People of the North feel an almost innate duty to strive for development, personal growth, and maturation. However, people without the North should not be seen as lethargic when they oppose changes; they are not trying to avoid hard work. They are sometimes merely oblivious to certain needs and requirements of the moment, or do not recognize them until it is too late.

The people without the North have many tasks to complete within themselves and with the world. When everything goes well, they think it is too good to last. It is far more difficult to compensate for the absence of the North than for the absence of any other Number combination or Station. It is even possible that people whose North is not occupied might not like reading this book. New perspectives of this type are not always the intellectual and spiritual nourishment that these people crave.

How can we perform some "first aid" in this case? What can you do when you consciously feel the absence of the North in your date of birth? It is essential for those who are missing the ❻ and ❶ to make a conscious effort to work with the color blue because a person with a missing North can often forget the vital regeneration phases and pauses. In this case, we recommend an old method. Write ❻ and ❶ on a blue piece of paper and carry it around with you, or secretly slip it to other people who could benefit from it. In earlier times, this method was commonly used to heal people because it worked without the knowledge or the faith of the recipients.

Blue or black clothing offers support through the colors' protective qualities. They shield us from external influences and assist in self-reflection. For someone without the North, this is difficult yet so important. "Airheads," who keep doing foolish things, can be brought back down to earth by blue and black. If you know someone who has an empty North and you would like to help this person along, it would be beneficial to have strong proof for your recommendations. Scientists who do not have the ❻ and ❶ in their birthdate sometimes suffer gladly since they tend to stubbornly insist on their own points of view, even when confronted with science that could soften their stance.

By the way, your Zodiac sign has an influence on the consequences of your Numbers. It can intensify, hamper, or complete their effect, and can also fill gaps. If you were born under a creative water sign (Cancer, Scorpio, or Pisces), then nothing will stand in the way of your having a career as a journalist, even if your North is missing.

We hope that we were able to bring the Numbers of the North to life. Going forward, whether you have these Numbers or not, you now have the tools to work on your life tasks.

Medicine for the Soul

Like every flower wilts, like each youth
yields to age, so each stage blossoms.
Each wisdom and each virtue flowers
in its own time, and must not last forever.
The heart must, at each new call for life,
be prepared for farewell and a fresh start.
To merge with courage and without grief
into different and new ties and bonds.
In each beginning, there dwells a special magic
that protects us and helps us to live.

—Hermann Hesse
(translated by Thomas Poppe)

Even animals of the same kind—two deer, two owls—will behave differently from each other. Even your daughter's own little pet hamsters; they all have their own ways. I have studied many plants. The leaves of one plant, on the same stem—none is exactly alike. On all the earth, there is not one leaf that is exactly like another. The Great Spirit, Wakan Tanka, likes it that way. He only sketches out the path of life roughly for all the creatures on earth, shows them where to go, where to arrive at, but leaves them to find their own way to get there. He wants them to act independently, according to their own nature, to the urges in each of them.

—Lame Deer

Happiness is not having what you want. It is wanting what you have.

—Anonymous
(*translated by Thomas Poppe*)

4

The East (❽ and ❸)

Empathy and Clarity of Vision

The People of the East: The Gift of the ❽ and/or ❸ in Your Birthdate

Those who can clearly see through people and things—those who are not deceived by a pretty facade—almost always have the ❽ or ❸ in their date of birth. This unmistakable characteristic, with the added ability to react correctly and in a timely fashion, was not given to everyone at birth. Many must work hard for it. The people of the East, on the other hand, are masters at avoiding *faux pas*. They were born with the natural instinct to do the right thing at the right time. Rejoice if you have the Numbers of the East as part of your date of birth. These Numbers present you with a built-in intuition.

With this strong empathy and your ability to sense the flow of energies, more doors will open for you than for others. You should accept this gift gratefully, and let it come to life. If you take care of it properly and keep it active, it will help you read people and situations correctly throughout your life. Anything is possible, from dealing with children to healing others to attaining musical perfection.

However, maintenance is important. Like any other ability, whether innate or acquired, it has to be kept active. And maintenance is best done by conscious use; if we do not take care of and sharpen our senses by using our talents and gifts, we will slowly turn blind, deaf, and mute. Our sensitivity will suffer and dwindle.

Every action and every thought have consequences, whether we are aware of them or not. For people with the East in their Code, the ❽ or ❸ equip them from the beginning with the ability to see the consequences of what they set into motion by thought or by deed; they are born with the ability to think things through to their conclusion. This includes judging where a billiard ball will roll and what will follow after a chess move, and if they want to (and have not learned early on to put their heads in the sand), people with ❽ or ❸ in their date of birth are able to look beyond the obvious to see the fire of reality behind the smokescreen of advertising propaganda.

One of the reasons they are natural healers is they are not misled by symptoms. They see the causes clearly. Many people of the East do not waste time in the study of conventional medicine and its focus on symptoms; they intuitively know that understanding and treating the cause, not the symptom, is the best path for healing. They will be the ones to lead the return to this holistic approach.

Shortly after World War I, a young Romanian physician was working in one of many overcrowded orphanages of Europe when he noticed that babies in a certain ward appeared to be more cheerful and lively. They also seemed to be better nourished and were ill less often than other children in their age group. He was immediately convinced that someone was feeding these children additional meals. After a while, however, he realized there was only one difference: the caretaker of these children made the effort to lift each child out of bed to cuddle him or her before feeding and putting the child back into his or her crib.

People with the ❽ or ❸ in their date of birth would be the types to give attention to the babies like this; this is the ❽ and ❸ in action. People of the East are going to be the ones who, in the near future, show modern medicine how to connect the dots, putting an end to the fiddling around with symptoms instead of learning about real causes and real cures.

Like all Numbers in one's birthdate, the Numbers of the East also confer a special responsibility to their owners. People of the East receive the power of empathy, both in the context of their own small world and in the larger world. They also gain the ability and perseverance to fight for a cause, even if it takes a long time.

Their "medicine cabinet" for the soul contains a rare ingredient, and this ingredient keeps them from being dependent upon instant success or tied to a foreseeable end result. They have the ability to take a stand for what is right, even though they may not live to see the happy outcome. In addition, people of the East have the ability to persevere, even when things become uncomfortable and the longed-for rest is nowhere in sight.

Martin Luther, the founder of Lutheranism, was born with the Numbers ❶❶/❶0/14❽❸. Luther said, "Even if I knew that tomorrow the world would go to pieces, I would still plant my apple tree."

The East is the home of vision, and vision enables us to understand situations that we have not experienced personally. Youthful energy will also be present with those in the East to a ripe old age, as the hope that we can accomplish something good is never abandoned. This same energy that young people use to conquer the world is also natural and profitable for the ❽ and ❸.

Sometimes, we relinquish all of these qualities, perhaps letting go voluntarily because we are afraid of life, or because using these abilities might become uncomfortable. Or we may let go involuntarily because we were suppressed by an environment that could not deal with the truth. You say you don't feel the special powers of the East even though you have an ❽ or ❸ in your date of birth? We promise that you will—*just not yet!*

One of the big challenges of the East lies in the gap between intuition and action; between a correct perception and its consequence lies the correct action. It often happens in life that correct perception does not lead to correct implementation, and complacency—even downright laziness— are definitely present in the East. Many bearers of the ❽ or ❸ are content with their precise emotions, calmly regarding everything from a distance. After a while, there is a rude awakening, and the East is surprised that the result is unpleasant. After all, everything had been so beautiful! The ❽ and ❸ forget at times that correct perception without correct action is like refusing to open a Christmas present because the anticipation may be more enjoyable than the present itself.

It is strange but true that many people are aware of what would be the right thing to do and are convinced that this insight is somehow valuable, even if they don't act upon it. For example, they might say, "I know how a good teacher should act to defend my children." But then they take no action when their children are being bullied in school. Or they may act like the know-it-all of political wisdom but fail to apply these insights in their everyday life. The only thing that can free us from this vicious cycle of complacency is willpower and the realization that even climbing Mount Everest begins with one small step. It is never too late to get going and take action.

After the description of the powers of the East, it comes as no surprise that the ❽ and ❸ tend to govern professions and fields in social, people-oriented areas, where the talents of the East blossom. The spectrum ranges from healers and physicians to caregivers, psychologists, preachers, singers, and musicians. As skillful and patient negotiators, they are generally in the professions that require a lot of patience, like organic farming and animal keeping, teaching, and so on.

In this context, the fine difference between the Numbers sometimes comes into play. The ❸ has a slightly greater tendency toward being a physician and healer, while the ❽ carries with it a slightly stronger draw toward musical energy.

The people of the East can be quite refreshing because they always have something planned. The East represents a new external beginning, as well as revival. It also represents spring, which is why it is associated with the color green; green moves things ahead and developments take place more quickly. Wherever something gets bogged down, people of the East will come to help because they love challenges. And everyone is happy when they appear, because their likeable demeanor and their gentle actions make all true collaboration easier. Patience is simply one of the built-in tools of the ❽ and ❸. One of their favorite jobs is to remove the monkey wrench from the machinery of any circumstance in life.

Children of the East

Children with the ❽ or ❸ in their date of birth show a high degree of sensitivity from an early age. When raising these children, it is important to never leave them alone without their knowledge. Although they can be left alone without a problem, these children neither forget nor easily forgive when they are disappointed or lied to, albeit with the best intentions. It shakes their belief in the world right down to its foundation. You are unlikely to regain their trust immediately just by saying, "Sorry, I meant well."

These children should not hear or see scary stories before going to bed (classic fairy tales belong to this category also). These stories keep them from falling asleep for a long time and follow them into their dreams. Harry Potter as a bedtime treat? Not a good idea for children of the East! Generally, children with an ❽ or ❸ take things very much to heart. They are deep thinkers and sometimes go through life (and school) in a dream-like way, spending a lot of time in thought.

How can we encourage children who have the ❽ or ❸? We should provide much affection, attention, patience, and understanding. We should also support their artistic talents by letting them learn musical instruments and by encouraging their natural abilities. That in itself is a guarantee that their special talents will be able to unfold.

◆ ◆ A Story from Johanna ◆ ◆

During one of my seminars, a farmer's wife mentioned her family's problems with the intended transfer of their farm to their son. Their seventeen-year-old son was passionate about his music lessons. Even as a ten-year-old, he had wanted a piano, and he had big problems with the idea of having to take over the farm. The family was worried as to how this would work out. The farmer's wife was relieved to hear about the Code, which put everything in a different light. We found out that the son had an ❽ and a ❸, which was ideal for a career in music. And there was something else: they had a four-year-old daughter who, from the time she could walk, spent a lot of time in the barn, helping wherever she could and even handling oversized pitchforks. Lo and behold, the daughter had both the ⓪ and ⑤ in her date of birth—ideal Numbers for closeness to nature and farming. The farmer's wife said, "Now I am going home, and we are going to buy our son his piano. And then we can relax and wait for our daughter to be ready to take over the farm."

Shadows on the East: The Promise Not Yet Fulfilled

What happens when your date of birth contains an ⑧ or ⑧ but you don't recognize yourself in the Numbers of the East? What if someone you know has these Numbers but shows little trace of the abilities we describe?

Not to worry. There are surely reasons why things developed this way. All it takes is a close look at the childhood events that prevented the treasure chest from opening completely. Whatever might have happened, it is never too late to accept your gift and turn it into a source of strength. It is your life and your story; you should never allow others to take over the writing of your script.

Perhaps you started keeping your true feelings to yourself very early in life because no one in your family understood them. Maybe it is part of your family traditions to simply not show emotions, so you have become accustomed to keeping them to yourself. This may even have been reinforced by harmful and false phrases like "Real men don't cry." (We believe that this miserable saying from sad times has even caused wars, because nothing is further from the truth. It is obvious that real men are not only quite capable of crying and showing emotions but it is in these times that they truly deserve to be called "real.")

Virtually all bad habits can be traced to the suppression of feelings—to the instilled inability to get to know them, name them, and own them. This is especially important when it comes to a healthy way of dealing with love and sexuality. Why is it that we watch hundreds of murders on television every day but rarely see a beautiful, heartfelt love scene without pornographic overtones? If you meditate on this question and wisely integrate the answers you find into your life, you will have taken a big step forward.

Try to discover your personal reasons for numbing your East. If you do not recognize yourself in the description of the East but are truly happy with your current state, then you have no reason to dwell on this very long. You have merely arranged your life differently, and that is just fine.

Should you feel, however, that your East is merely in hiding and would like to come to life, there are a number of ways can awaken it. Working with colors is the simplest and quickest way to do this. Whether in your wardrobe, house, office, bedroom, living room, children's rooms, carpets, drapes, pictures, or linens—the only limit is your imagination. Since green is the color of the East, wear as much green as possible to awaken this Station. If green is already your favorite color, you are intuitively on the right road. (But be careful: if you are a truly actualized person of the East, you do not need that much green.) Additionally, in order to bring out the energy of the East, you should have greens in your diet, including vegetables, salads, and herbs.

If what you have read so far makes you realize that you are in the wrong profession, then you might want to think about engaging in hobbies and activities that provide new nourishment for you in the East. Fortunately, the musical talent of the ❽ and ❸ can be taken up at any time and can give you a lot of inner contentment; you do not have to go as far as forming a band to revitalize the East. Just try approaching music intuitively, doing whatever feels right.

Another simple and effective method of awakening the East consists of writing the Numbers ❽ and ❸ on a small piece of paper and carrying them around. (Green paper will strengthen the effect.) You might shake your head at this and think, "How can something like that help?" Admittedly, it does sound somewhat outlandish. However, many things in this world cannot be explained, but they still work beautifully. Imagine if a baby first asks for proof that mother's milk is healthy before the child accepts this source of nourishment?

Essentially, we are offering a little "mother's milk" here. And its greatest health value can only be obtained by drinking it, so try it out. Find out how well everything functions. Do not allow anyone to deprive you of the enormous power of your personal experience—not well-meaning experts or anyone else who prefers scientific proof to healthy common sense. If the former were in charge, the world would be in worse condition than it already is. The Code can help you find the way back to the joyous and loving plan that was intended for you.

Awakening the East's "green" abilities in your Wheel brings out the best in you, thereby contributing to the well-being of all the people around you. And when someone teases you by saying, "I've never seen this side of you," then simply smile to yourself and know that you are on the right track.

Do not let anyone take your progress away. Those who care about you accept you as you are. They are happy about your every development, movement, and awakening. Only those who want to exploit your good nature would stand to benefit if nothing were to change, and you need not enable their selfishness any longer. Consider that you are teaching them a valuable lesson by allowing your quiet assurance to bring forth their egotism.

When the East Needs Taming: Development into the Extreme

What happens when the deep-reaching energies (in the truest sense of the word) get out of hand and become overpowering? This occurs mostly when there are too many Units of the ❽ or ❸ in your birthdate—dates like August 3, 1988, or March 18, 1938. Quite often, an abundance of these Numbers in this Cardinal Point is too much of a good thing. Extremely sensitive people like these tend to hide their feelings and observations rather than learning how to deal with the powerful energies that could lead them in a fruitful direction. These people are likely to suppress feelings and insights whose actualization might generate a shift in family or community dynamics.

At times, extreme people from the East might actually come across as distant because their highly developed empathy and perceptions overwhelm them and push them into a standoffish silence. Their well-meaning contemporaries sometimes have problems dealing with them as well because they intuitively know that these people are not who they appear to be.

Professionally, an overdeveloped ❽ or ❸ can lead to the absentminded professor syndrome. An example of this would be the musical genius who needs someone to bring his sheet music to the concert hall, or needs to be reminded that slippers don't go with a tuxedo and a concert performance. There are more examples like this, but you surely know what kind of people we are talking about. These people will always need to overcome "the shadow of the East" and actively strive for more discipline to avoid getting lost in day-to-day life.

The extreme can also move in the other direction. People with a strong East often appear overly empathetic and superhumanly patient—almost too good to be true. But on the inside, they are ready to explode. These walking powder kegs need an outlet for their pent-up emotions, and unfortunately, their own family often ends up becoming their emotional lightning rod or trash can.

Consequently, it is also possible that people of the East will end up feeling constantly used, and justifiably so. They tend to be suddenly resistant, much to the surprise of those around them. In order to successfully tame the excessive energies of the East, it is crucial to create a more controlled outlet for emotions to prevent them from offending others. Living together becomes much easier with planning, scheduling, good daily organization, and deliberate action.

Those who feel a heavily weighted East should avoid wearing green clothing and act cautiously on particular days and dates that contain the ❽ or ❸. When the goal is the neutralization or healing of an extreme over-development, the colors of the opposite Station can be helpful. In the case of the East, it would be the color of the West, namely, white. If your West is missing, surrounding yourself with people who have the Numbers of the West (❾ or ❹) will also be helpful.

Further, in order to derive the biggest benefit from our Numbers gift, we should pass our treasure clockwise around the circle to the next Station. In the case of the East, that would be the South, to people with the ❼ or ❷, who will enthusiastically promote the good ideas of the East.

Now you know where your talents lie as a person of the East. It does not matter if your treasures are waiting to be exposed or if your energies need taming. Let your true abilities show, and you will be happy.

When the East Is Missing: The Birthdate without the ❽ and/or ❸

Imagine someone is walking toward you on the street. There is plenty of room for everybody, but this person wants to pass in the exact spot where you are standing and you end up blocking each other. Or imagine a flow of people using a revolving door or a flight of stairs: everything is rolling smoothly until someone stops moving to consult a map. Anyone who does this almost certainly does not have the Numbers of the East in his or her birthdate. When you have the ❽ or ❸ in your date of birth, you have so much instinct and feeling that it is unlikely you would become the "offender" described above.

People without the ❸ in their date of birth cannot stand a lot of commotion; without the ❽, they are likely to deal with things in a complicated way because the natural, organic approach that would quickly pick up on existing energy flows is missing. Although having musical talent is as natural to the East as the dawn, there are still many musical people whose date of birth does not contain an ❽ or ❸. They sometimes do not have enough feeling for correct measure, beat, and musical cue but are capable of learning those over time. Having been an obstacle to the multiple flows in everyday life acts as a powerful inspiration to fill an empty East!

There are a number of ways to fill the voids in your life and in your Wheel. As with all empty Stations, the best path is to first work with the associated color. We've talked about how you can put a small piece of green paper with the Numbers ❽ and ❸ written on it in your purse or pocket. A small piece of green material in your pocket will help, too, even if there are no Numbers written on it. It does not have to be something obtrusive. (You have probably guessed by now why you have always liked green a lot.)

When the ❽ and the ❸ are missing, the body simply needs more green—something you can compensate for by adding more green food to your diet. In earlier times, people paid close attention to color connections by working with stones. This is effective because a stone can accompany you anywhere, and you can buy several for your purse, briefcase, pockets, nightstand, office, kitchen, living room, and so on. To radiate the energy of the East, use green stones decoratively in water-filled glass decanters or directly on the soil of flowerpots.

Perhaps the most important step in the conquest of the East is to learn to listen better in conversation until you comprehend what your counter-part really means, even beyond what is expressed in words. The people of the East already possess this ability, but they must consciously develop it. And this is feasible!

People with an empty East (or with too much East) have a tendency to say what they do not mean. They do not always feel empathy regarding the effects and consequences of what they put out into the world. Only when you dare to feel this lack (and it is important to do so without self-recrimination) will you be able to fill this void in the East more quickly.

As we said earlier in discussing the Wheel's spiral movement, a gener-ally valid and successful way to fill voids is to share your work, thoughts, ideas, suggestions, and intentions with other people. This transfer ensures that your energies do not lose momentum and that the Wheel continues to turn. This means that a lively development takes place. (At this point, you might want to read once more the chapter about the Wheel's spiral move-ment on page 13.)

Sometimes people without the ❽ or ❸ in their birthdate avoid people of the East—of all people! We say "of all people" because they are the best ones to help you fill the void. The reason for this is simple: you often per-ceive these people as being "too emotional" because you neither speak much about your own feelings nor do you usually have the urge. This might sound a bit harsh, but in no case does it mean that people without the ❽ or the ❸ in their date of birth are emotionally cold. They simply do not make a big fuss about their feelings.

Herein lies the key: mostly, it is enough to understand the East. When you, not having the East, show more emotion, you will have taken a big step, to the delight of those around you. You do not have to do much more in order to see positive changes and more happiness in your life. And the whole world will benefit!

Medicine for the Soul

Softness triumphs over hardness, feebleness over strength.
What is more malleable is always superior over that which is immovable.
This is the principle of controlling things by going along with them,
Of mastery through adaptation.

—Lao Tzu

Trusting in God is the key to happiness.
But without taking things into your own hand, it is incomplete.
When the beard catches fire, it is not very smart to pray for rain.

—**Paramahansa Yogananda**

5

The South (❼ and ❷)

Fire and Passion

The People of the South: The Gift of the ❼ and/or ❷ in Your Birthdate

It is clear that when you have received the gift of the ❼ or ❷ in your date of birth, a vibrant personality is your birthright. It is difficult to escape the spell of your charisma, and one should not even try.

People of the South come across as being strong, expressive, and energetic. They offer the world the proverbial strong shoulder to lean on, and it seems like they are able to accomplish anything. But beware; they do not always deliver what they promise. This is a consequence of periodic or chronic overload rather than a lack of power.

People who are curious and passionate also have the ❼ or ❷ as part of their date of birth. They exude curiosity and cheerfulness early in the morning, which can be difficult to tolerate for anyone who is not a morning person. As adults, these people like variety and are not homebodies. Although they are thrifty, they get a lot of projects up and running, and in so doing, a tendency toward extravagance might manifest itself. This does not automatically happen, however, and is more of a concern when the Center of Gravity is in the South.

The season of the South, of the ❼ and ❷, is summer. It is the joyful maturation process where experiences become realized—the high point of life, when peaches are ripe on the trees. It should come as no surprise then that the vibrant color red is assigned to this Cardinal Point of the Birthday Wheel.

As far as the difference in strength goes, there is only a minimal gradation between the ❼ and the ❷. The ❷ is fiercer, more spontaneous, and less enduring. The ❼ imparts a little more personality but does not act as spontaneously, taking longer while being somewhat more enduring.

The charismatic aura of the people of the South can literally fill a room, and it usually feels good to work alongside them. They almost always find quick solutions to problems and are strangers to lengthy brooding. People of the South are also entertaining and enjoyable companions.

Philosophers, architects, researchers, and painters can easily befriend the South and its characteristics. When priests preach convincingly, it is frequently due to a ❼ or ❷ in their date of birth. However, when a public speaker is missing the South, they can be difficult to listen to. Without the strong characters of theater, film, and television from the South, the entire world of media would be poorer. Without the presence of the ❼ and ❷, revolutionaries of all types would have difficulty finding comrades-in-arms to help fight for their cause. Monks with their extreme way of life also belong to the South, their apparent tranquility notwithstanding.

People of the South always find an attentive audience. No matter how good a politician might be, without a ❼ or ❷ in his or her date of birth, election season will be a difficult time. This void brings with it the hidden danger of superficial, inflammatory rhetoric that can cause a great deal of damage. People without willpower, without the ability to discriminate, without personal responsibility—all fall prey to convincing speakers; many irrational persecutions began with a convincing spokesperson. This is why many a windbag or pitchman can be found with a ❼ or ❷, unless other Cardinal Points or life experiences provide a balance.

The energy of the ❼ or ❷ ensures the ability to tackle difficult tasks and also provides enormous perseverance along the way. An idea does not evaporate in a few days, even if everything doesn't go as planned. It is thanks to people with these Numbers that serious violations get reported and dark machinations are uncovered. But perseverance has to be worthwhile! In the eyes of the people of the South, perseverance without the prospect of success is not rewarding.

Children of the South

For children with a ❼ or ❷ in their date of birth, it is a good idea for them to play and get their energy out before going to sleep. They become almost ill if they get the feeling that they have not fully taken advantage of the day. (Counting sheep will not help them.) The ❼ and ❷ create the desire to experience and conquer life, and bookworms are rarely found under Signatures where the South is the Center of Gravity.

A birthday party without children of the South can be dreadfully dull, which is why introverted people usually find these children to be exhausting. It would be best to encourage children of the South to play sports so that they have an outlet for their energy. They love challenges and enjoy the external recognition of trophies and medals. They are also natural competitors who like to be the center of attention—especially when awards are being handed out. Many kids enjoy hiking, but children of the South expect a merit badge when they get done. Otherwise it would not have been worthwhile.

There is a danger here: if this need for recognition persists into adulthood, there is a tendency to be easily manipulated. We all know people who would give everything for a tin trophy. Unfortunately, they are likely to be on their own when it comes to overcoming such childishness since these tendencies are exploited and encouraged in many areas of adult life. "Employee of the Month" awards are an example of such pittances.

Danger recognized is danger vanquished. When children of the South display tendencies like this, praise them, but teach them at the same time the difference between true approval and stick-and-carrot incentives. Children are quick learners and will be able to detect hypocrisy more easily as adults with your guidance now.

Shadows on the South: The Promise Not Yet Fulfilled

Let's assume you know a corpulent couch potato who has the ❼ or ❷ in his or her date of birth but whose description in no way fits the Numbers of the South. What happened to this person?

The energy of the South is plentiful but loses its shining power when it encounters choking, darkening energies. Expressions like "Don't do that!" or "Leave that alone!" or "Be careful!" or "Stop making such a fuss!" are often accompanied by stern measures to enforce parental authority. When a cheerful disposition and the passion of the South are constantly being suppressed, this can lead to resigned idleness and sometimes unchecked, violent outbursts.

For many centuries, such conditions have been misused for self-serving purposes. Whenever someone's innate joyfulness and enthusiasm is suppressed, it is much easier to control him or her with a promise of a distant joy for malicious purposes. All indoctrination and brainwashing thrive on this process.

People who have learned to cover the South must look deep into themselves in order to revive the energy of the ❼ and ❷. It might be necessary to ask for outside help, possibly in the form of "family constellation therapy." This is a fairly recent discovery that has developed into one of the most effective, deep-reaching tools available for bringing light to what has been forgotten or suppressed.

We recommend this treatment for people who do not recognize themselves in their Numbers. In most cases, their developmental flow was interrupted during childhood or earlier in their family history, inhibiting or blocking the maturation process to self-actualization. The chubby couch potato who has the Numbers of the South has a lid on his or her true destiny and life energy. Being overweight is often the sea anchor that was tossed out by the soul in order to slow down the body-ship and obscure the true energy of the captain.

Do not be discouraged! This shyness is short-lived, but the joy and insight in the newly won freedom are long-term. An experienced therapist can get things moving in the right direction. (You can find a list of qualified family constellation therapists at www.hellinger.com or by searching the internet for "family constellation therapy.")

If your South is covered in shadows, revitalization is crucial. As of now, start wearing more red clothing. Go to parties and experience life again—it belongs to you. Of course, there are stages in life when we do not feel like doing those very things, and that is absolutely fine! Many situations require time for handling and digesting, for grieving and adjusting. There is a time for everything in life, including awakening. If you have taken your frustration to the living room couch and use television programs and junk food to numb your ability to feel and to think, then you are doing something wrong. Having the South in your Wheel, you fall into the group of courageous people who have the ability to bounce back no matter what gets them down in life. One of your life's tasks is to embody this resilient quality as a role model for others. If the South is in hiding, there is usually a reason for it. Bring it out into the light, and everything will fall into place again.

More often than not, a strong personality is responsible for the suppression of the ❼ or ❷. But what is your real reason for submitting to it? Maybe you have never thought about it in depth. Is someone standing behind you with a weapon, forcing you to do what you are doing? If you defend yourself, your tormentor might just be left flabbergasted.

◆　◆　◆　◆　◆

Seemingly quiet and laid-back people (when the fire and charisma of the South are hidden) are sitting on an emotional powder keg. They have been taught behavioral and thinking patterns that will prevent anyone from knowing how they actually feel. This is not only dangerous but can lead to chronic illness. If no one knows your true feelings, then you are constantly collecting blasting powder, ounce by ounce.

Once in a while, some of the people of the South take a vacation alone where no one knows them. Lo and behold, we would not recognize them in the hustle and bustle into which they throw themselves or which they initiate. It is the right thing to do; valves must be opened. Learn a healthy way to deal with your energies as soon as possible. The sooner you find a positive way to channel them, the less you need to let off external steam abruptly or be internally destructive. It is perfectly acceptable to practice on strangers. Little by little, you will live your life in the way it was meant to be lived, according to your temperament. You should not hide yourself away. Always remember that every person has the right to be accepted, welcomed, and loved.

When the South Needs Taming: Development into the Extreme

All Cardinal Points are subject to overdevelopment, especially when more than ten Units are present (this would be the case when the ❼ appears twice). In the South, however, a formation of such a Center of Gravity is even more extreme, because its manifestation is more dramatic. If this development takes place in the East (❽/❸), it might not be noticed for a long time because it often manifests as deep emotional withdrawal. With the South, you can more quickly recognize the danger when temperament escalates to overexcitability and enthusiasm turns into hysterics. There is also the danger of sliding into a sudden wrath, domineering behavior, or bossiness. Fortunately, it is easy to control the extreme with simple means, but it is always a personal decision.

Children who have the South as their Center of Gravity should not be constantly curbed or rebuked. Instead, their energies should be channeled into sensible activities. Their need to be physically active would be best served in sports, where the child will surely leave every competitor in the dust. Not everyone has the endurance for sports, but it is definitely present in the strong South. And then there is dancing. The ability to dance was given to them at birth. Of course, everyone can dance, and it would be a true step forward for mankind if dancing became a part of the standard school curriculum. The children of the South do not need to learn how to dance, though. For the most part, they understand dancing already; they just need to learn the steps, and they are off. While others drag themselves across the dance floor, gasping for air, children of the South lightheartedly float past them, even if the South's history includes an addiction to television and junk food.

Children with many ❼s or ❷s in their date of birth should not eat cooked food too often in the evening. It is best to give them none, as they will find it difficult to sleep. The cooking process endows food with the invisible energy of the color red, thus increasing red's strength. (However, if a child is missing the South, cooked porridge or warm soup is the perfect thing to make him or her sleepy.) Those whose South shows more than ten Units should also avoid wearing red and be more cautious on days when the date contains a ❼ and/or ❷.

By the way, observing the rules of the Code would surely be a blessing for fashion designers. When choosing the "color of the year" for their upcoming collections, they should observe the Cardinal Point's colors. In other words, when the fourth digit of the year is a ❼ or ❷, it would be wise to declare red among the fashionable colors of that year. The same goes for green when the fourth digit of the year ends with ❽ or ❸, for yellow when ⓪ or ⑤ are present, for blue or black in years with ❻ or ❶, and for white in years with ❾ or ❹. Sometimes, designers take note of a given year's preference in the unconscious buying habits of customers and try to repeat that success in the coming year. Then—surprise!—the fad is gone. And you now know why.

When an extreme development needs to be neutralized or healed, the color of the opposite Station can be helpful. In the case of the South, it would be the color of the North, namely, blue or black. It can be quite helpful to surround yourself with people whose birthdate contains a ❻ or ❶, especially when you have no North. The highest success rate is possible when we pass our treasure around the circle to the next Station. In the case of the South, this would pass to the West—to people who have a ❾ or ❹ in their date of birth. This will immediately provide the tools to tame the extreme South.

❖ ❖ A Story from Johanna ❖ ❖

I sometimes conduct "Moon Weeks," which are seminars about natural and lunar rhythms, and many other aspects of the ancient knowledge we lived by on our farm. A few years ago, I briefly introduced the Code during one of those seminars to see if the time was ripe for it. One of the participants covered her face with her hands, and sat there pale and miserable. I asked her afterward if I had insulted her. (This can happen when we first reveal the Code.) She responded aghast, "I'm crushed. For years, I have been telling my daughter to wear more red. I even bought her red things for her apartment because she is always tired and downcast. Now I find out that with two ❼s in her date of birth, she is hopelessly overwhelmed with the South and red." This woman was, of course, not aware of the Code and its intricate connections, but everything turned out fine. The daughter is doing well and even belatedly graduated from high school (wearing mostly blue clothes).

Finally, one more suggestion. People with a heavily occupied South tend to perspire more than others. If they do not, in order to compensate, they get a fever faster than other people. Taking a vacation in a hot climate without having cooling water from a beach or a pool as balance totally exhausts them. The coolness of the mountains, however, balances the warmth in their temperament. Blue skies and mild temperatures are the thing of dreams for people of the South. A blue and black wardrobe cools their temperament to a level that is also pleasant for them.

When the South Is Missing: The Birthdate without the ❼ and/or ❷

When, after all you have read, you take a look at your birthdate and are disappointed that it does not contain a ❼ or ❷, have courage. Help is on the way! You only need to realize that your tasks and talents lie elsewhere. Of course, it is part of our basic makeup to feel the voids in your Code and want to do something about it. Not only is this acceptable, it is even our task in life. You do not have to become like a person of the South, however; it is sufficient to simply understand the South.

Some people do not feel this need and then do not know why they don't have an overall feeling of well-being. People with a ❼ or ❷ will always find an attentive audience. People without the South often feel mis-understood and unappreciated, no matter how well they express themselves or how great their external influence actually is. Even during a run of suc-cess, there is always a spark of fear present. As an aside, if you were born under a fire sign (Aries, Leo, or Sagittarius), it is possible that you might not feel the absence of the South very much.

What advice do we have for you if you consciously feel the missing South? Let's start with colors. The color red in all its shades can bring you more strength and energy that you might otherwise miss when things become "serious." Maybe you have good ideas but do not have the strength to convey them? Maybe you often feel overlooked, no matter how good you are? There are many reasons why a person might sometimes feel left out. From now on, you can counteract that by filling your empty South.

One good way of doing this is to spend a lot of time outside in the sun (with the necessary sun protection, of course). Learn to love the day, not just the evening! In the evening, you can work with candles and tea lights glowing in red glass holders. When you experience that empty feeling, listen to lively music instead of meditative notes. Little things like that can save the day! Although visiting a museum is highly uplifting and educa-tional, a good movie is sometimes better for the mind—just as playing music yourself to get your circulation going is better than drinking a lot of coffee.

It would probably take a few years or a few centuries to describe why this works. Today, it is only important to know that it does. Write the Numbers ❼ and ❷ on a small piece of red paper and carry them around in your purse or pocket. Give it a try; you have nothing to lose. When it comes to food, there are also a number of ways to replace the ❼ and ❷. From now on, eat red apples instead of green ones, drink red grape juice instead of white, and have a glass of red wine instead of white.

The fairness of the universe also ensures that the negative sides of the ❼ and ❷ do not affect you. Everything has a positive side. Reread the chapter that covers the Numbers that appear in your date of birth, and make the very best of the information. Incorporate into your life the ideas we presented to fill the void in your South.

Small changes on a daily basis are much more effective in changing the world than doing something big every now and then.

Medicine for the Soul

He who sows a thought today
Will harvest the deed tomorrow,
Then a habit the day after,
Then the character,
And finally his fate.
Therefore, he needs to meditate upon
What he sows today.
And needs to understand,
That his fate is in his own hands: Today!

—**Gottfried Keller**
(***translated by Thomas Poppe***)

I have never done marketing.
I simply loved my clients.

—**Zino Davidoff**

All good things in the world come directly from our soul.
All bad things in the world come from the fog
That enshrouds our soul.
Wander through the fog until it lifts.
Don't stop wandering, you will reach your destination.
Is there a shortcut? Yes, there is.
It is the realization that we create the fog ourselves.

—**Ron Fischer**

6

The West (❾ and ❹)

Skill and Prudence

The People of the West: The Gift of the ❾ and/or ❹ in Your Birthdate

The West, with the ❾ or ❹ in your date of birth, infuses life with tremendous strength. One could say that those who find a ❾ (but not the ❾ found in 1900!) have pretty much won. For mere mortals who do not have the bonus of the ❾, dealing with these strong people is not always easy. In truth, those with a ❾ usually get their way. Although people who do not know what they want in life are generally more difficult to bear, the determination and efficiency of the people of the West, especially those with a ❾, can get on your last nerve. Remember, we can only do the best for all concerned if we are able to put ourselves into the other person's shoes. This is important in daily life and for getting along with others.

Do you have the West in your date of birth? People with the ❾ or ❹ are not just successful in theory but are also prepared to be very hard working, and at times extremely industrious. Your ambition and drive to succeed put you at the forefront.

Your "creative phase" tends to last a lifetime. You rarely close your ears to constructive criticism, especially when it will bring you something new and result in meaningful changes. Your inborn ambition combined with your prudence puts you among the front-runners. It is rare to find a boss, manager, chief executive officer, or attorney who does not have a ❾ or ❹ in his or her birthdate.

Highly skilled craftsmen are also at home in the West. People of the West frequently feel most comfortable in professions that allow them to create, build, or erect something, preferably with their own two hands. And it is almost always a pleasure to see these hands at work. When West hands dance, everyone else looks like they have two thumbs. It is sad to see how these skilled trades have lost prestige in contrast to purely academic professions. We can read about the consequences of this every day in the economic and environmental sections of our daily newspaper. We are happily looking forward to the day when someone can say, "I am a carpenter," and is met with great respect. We also look forward to the day when it becomes law that only those who have spent at least four years working in organic farming can become Secretary of Agriculture!

❖ ❖ A Story from Johanna ❖ ❖

A typical example for a healthy use of the Numbers ❾ and ❹ is evident in the comment made by a construction site manager. When I asked him what made his job so enjoyable, he replied, "I simply want to build something that will be here long after I am gone. Something tangible."

There were two other site managers present during this conversation. They were working on a large project, the construction of a highway viaduct. You could easily tell the people of the West; they were eagerly anticipating the completion of the bridge. Those without the West stood around looking bored. Being the company comptroller accountant at the time, I was surprised that so many people held the wrong positions. Construction companies should take a closer look at their two-thumbed workers to see if they have the West in their dates of birth and find them more suitable assignments. *What a blessing this knowledge would be for any human resource department, employment agency, or other similar business.*

The ❾ and ❹ provide perseverance and strong business acumen. The differences between the two Numbers with regard to business are minimal. Among people with a ❹, skilled workers, engineers, and do-it-yourselfers are more prevalent. Those with a ❾ tend to have a better business sense. Generally, people of the West are very demanding when choosing a profession. A run-of-the-mill job is out of the question for them unless they are forced to obtain one. They learn to astutely handle finances as naturally as a fish swims. It is almost as if the people of the West learn to calculate before they learn how to speak. Banking transactions are a daily pleasure for them, while they are more of a necessary evil for other Cardinal Points. This talent should definitely be put to work.

The West fears nothing and propels projects forward until they are completed. Brilliant inventors can also be found in the West. Sometimes their genius is way ahead of its time, and they only become famous posthumously. Engineers, financially savvy merchants, mechanics, pilots, race-car drivers, sports figures, and secretaries are all at home in the West. Competent office assistants and secretaries are often the heart and soul of a company—the backbones, motors, and reenergizers of successful top executives.

The power of the West, together with the energy of the ❾ and ❹, is part of the ideal makeup of these valuable people. You say you know such a pearl, but he or she does not have a ❾ or a ❹? Such exceptions are not that rare. Nothing in the world is really difficult, not even conquering the West. If, in addition to being determined, we are lucky enough to encounter a genuine, talented, and humane teacher, then this person can teach us how to enjoy effortlessly conquering the unknown West. We know several people without a ❾ or ❹ who have managed to master the number-heavy and fact-heavy materials of the West. Nothing is impossible.

Children of the West

In most cases, you do not have to train the children of the West; they will do as they please. This does not mean that they will inevitably become difficult children. On the contrary, they will live their lives in contentment as long as they are surrounded by good role models. The surest way to make life difficult for children with an emphasis in the West is to be a parent who always knows best.

Children of the West are fighters and winners! Give them the feeling that they can conquer new territory on their own. The expansive abilities inherent in the ❾ and ❹ provide a much easier start in life. Therefore, it is even more important to not hinder these children by neglecting or overtaxing them. Don't act like those silly souls who continuously uproot plants from flowerpots to see if the plants are rooting well. Children of the West can tolerate upheaval much less than children with other Cardinal Points.

On the other hand, Children of the West are often better able to fend off intervention into the development of their personality. A certain stubbornness or (better yet) tenacity will accompany them through life. This is a valuable trait as long as it stays within reasonable limits, so take their ambition seriously. Nothing would hurt them more than not being taken seriously and could result in aggressions that cannot be treated easily. When their pride is hurt, it can sometimes be permanent; as the more intelligent person, they feel it is beneath their dignity to make concessions. However, people of the West are also aware that this aggressive behavior only masks conflict avoidance and anxiety. Generally, they can sense the difference.

By now, you probably have gained a feel for the power and energy of the West. This power must be actualized, whether as a child or as an adult, as it is part of the legacy of the ❾ and ❹; money and riches are of great importance to the people of the West. And this wish in itself is not morally wrong. What counts is the intelligent and humanitarian management of your resources. It is part of what makes you happy in life.

Shadows on the West: The Promise Not Yet Fulfilled

Even though you have become better acquainted with the special powers of the ❾ and ❹, it is possible that you do not recognize yourself in this description or that you see it differently, despite having the West in your date of birth. If this holds true in your case or in the case of someone you know, then it is time to play "detective of the soul."

There are various reasons why the powers of the West might not fully blossom. If suppression began during early childhood and the sense of basic trust was lost, it will be more difficult to restore the flow with this blockage. The West imparts a great deal of purposefulness and willpower, but both of these characteristics can be driven out by an authoritarian upbringing. So many people know they have multiple abilities and attributes in them but simultaneously feel that they merely languish. Why not awaken them? Reading this book might just be enough to confirm in black and white what you've always known you have within you.

Perhaps it might be enough to awaken your memories and feelings of other times? It is imperative that you change your thinking here and now. Right now! Try it at least. Leave your old thought processes behind. Turn them off like an old movie of which you have seen enough. Write your own movie script! Then watch the new movie—and make sure you turn up the volume!

The color of the West is white. Work with the beneficial energy of this color every day to help you get into a good starting position. But only do this if it is truly your wish! If you do not recognize yourself in the description of the West (even with the ❾ or ❹ in your birthdate) but are truly happy with your life, then everything is good and you need not push to make changes. Assuming that you do want to change, however, you can gain a great deal just by using the color white in your clothing, in your home environment, and at your workplace. White makes you strong-willed, courageous, innovative, and self-assured, and living areas should display a lot of white. You should also severely limit the number of colorful knickknacks. White tablecloths are better for you than colored ones. Additionally, you should avoid wearing too much green. In this case, green contributes to blocking the energies of the West.

By using the ❾ and ❹ wisely in your daily life, a few things will be set in motion for you. Whenever possible, pick telephone Numbers, room Numbers, license plate Numbers, passwords, and so on that contain the

❾ or ❹. Writing the Numbers ❾ and ❹ on a white piece of paper or cloth and carrying it around also works well. Your intellect might balk a little, but that is fine; you do not have to be able to build a car before you can drive one. Above all, choose from our suggestions, but don't overdo it. The idea is only to awaken the West. Once the West is awake, everything can return to its correct proportions, including the emphasis on the color white in your life.

When the West Needs Taming: Development into the Extreme

When the West produces too much of a good thing, apply the opposite measures to those that activated the powers of the ❾ and/or ❹. It can happen that the concentration of a Cardinal Point needs balancing. If you have more than ten Units of the West in your date of birth, like April 16, 1969, then it is sometimes more difficult to deal with these powers.

An unhealthy overweighting of the West can manifest itself in egotistical outbursts, or by going it alone in your personal or business life in instances when only teamwork can lead to success. The ❾ provides a great deal of assertiveness, to the detriment of teamwork. Sound business sense can overdevelop to such a degree that it will exceed the limits of all that is human. The resulting materialism, corruption, and destructive energies will later destroy everything. As the psychologist Mihaly Csikszentmihalyi said, "A business activity that contributes nothing to human growth and well-being is not worth doing, independent of how large a profit it generates within a short period of time."

A hunger for power and selfishness can drive entire family businesses and companies to ruin. People with a ❾ often insist on having the last word in order to bolster their ego. Although this can also happen with other Cardinal Points, the danger is greater here.

For those who are not aware of the connection between the ❾ and ❹ and the color white, it is important to know the following: if they have been blessed with both Numbers, or they have the Number ❾ twice, wearing white will inadvertently strengthen the egotistical, willful tendencies of this combination. After all, two ❾s equals eighteen Units in the West, which is far above the ten-Unit threshold that signals the danger of going to extremes. In fact, people with this much weight in the West often have a difficult time tolerating hospitals because of the overload of white.

An overdeveloped West can also have the opposite effect. Instead of throwing themselves into cold, success-oriented business activities, these people can experience a type of intellectual paralysis—their minds capitulate when faced with an abundance of ideas, possibilities, and abilities. They have so many possibilities open to them that they do not know whether they are coming or going. This can be compared to a migraine headache, which is typically preceded by an overbooked schedule. It seems impossible to accomplish everything, so the mind goes blank.

These developments can be healed with the simplest means. If your West is strong, you should avoid wearing white, and act wisely by conserving your strength on dates that contain a ❾ or ❹. Take it step by step, and always tackle the most immediate and most closely related task. Do not squander your mental and physical strengths. The color of the opposite Station is always helpful in neutralizing and healing extremes. In the case of the West, it would be the color of the East, which is green. It is also quite productive to surround yourself with people whose date of birth contains the East (❽/❸), especially when you do not have the East yourself.

In order to enjoy the greatest benefit from a Station, you should not seal yourself off emotionally. Instead, pass your treasures around the circle to the next Station. In the case of the West, that would be to the North, to people with the ❻ or ❶ in their birthdate.

You can take action early enough but only after thinking it through. Do not rush things. (Patience is not exactly a virtue of the West.) You can intervene with the colors green and yellow in your home and work environment to regulate energies and open the door to harmony and balance. Taking things step by step is one of the best methods for counteracting an extreme overdevelopment in the West. Remember, slow and steady wins the race. Taking this saying to heart is the perfect remedy for the West, but it is up to you to pick the solutions that work well for you.

When the West Is Missing: The Birthdate without the ❾ and/or ❹

What can I do when my date of birth is missing the ❾ or ❹? How will I be able to develop the great talents that are inherent in the West? Does a missing ❹ mean that I have to accept having two left thumbs? Does a missing ❾ mean that I have to forgo working independently in my business life? Relax, it won't be as bad as that. Maybe you were lucky during your childhood and were allowed, when appropriate, to follow the natural instinct of all children, which is to fill any voids with enthusiasm.

If the above was not the case, have courage. First of all, it is not necessary to conquer and integrate the voids in your West; you only have to understand them. Second, we do not always miss what we do not have. People without the West in their date of birth do not have the industriousness and restlessness that are the very qualities that can make people of the West occasionally annoying. In addition, you will not be tempted to fall into the trap of the extreme overdevelopments of the West, which can definitely appear seductive.

In other words, a little insight into the West and its special qualities would not hurt anyone. Maybe this newly acquired knowledge will help you to see your daughter, whose date of birth contains a ❾ or ❹, as being less egotistical. Perhaps your father-in-law will appear less materialistic when you put aside your preconceived ideas that come from the other Cardinal Points of the Birthday Wheel. To start, just accept that the people of the West have different values in life. And who wants to appoint oneself as the judge who sets the rules?

◆ ◆ A Story from Johanna ◆ ◆

My personal date of birth contains neither a ❾ nor a ❹, and this surely influenced my decision to learn accounting as a young woman. I had the feeling that I needed this skill to be complete. I remember only too well how shocked I was when my boss said, "White is your favorite color, isn't it, Johanna?" The ❾ and ❹ are assigned to the color white, and the men -

tal qualities of the West (logical thinking, math skills, and organizational talent, among others) can be enhanced with white clothing. I felt caught and embarrassed. This shows just how secretive my family was when it came to the Code!

If you own a successful business without having a ❾ or ❹ in your date of birth, you have probably filled the voids in your West. You are therefore able to budget prudently so that your generosity does not put your company in the red. If you still find running a business tedious and tiresome, then consider taking on a colleague, partner, or assistant with the West in his or her birthdate to take over the finances or to run the office.

Be careful, however, not to have your own void exploited. Generally, people without the West need to budget their money carefully to avoid having their generosity taken advantage of. People without the West usually need a good watchdog, perhaps in the form of a tax adviser, who can show some teeth if necessary. Or maybe it would suffice to take a bookkeeping course in night school? When lacking this extra help, it is difficult to enjoy money and invest it wisely.

In order to conquer and integrate the West, you merely need to teach yourself financial foresight and sound economic thinking. You might want to reread "Shadows on the West" (see page 66), as the suggestions there are often enough to attract the qualities of the missing West, or to show you how to do well without them.

Make use of the guidance here to regularly beautify your day with added strength and energy. Consider white candles, white napkins on the table, and white in your clothes. Just trust your instincts, and after a while, your life will be much richer.

Medicine for the Soul

The new students on an Indian reservation frequently turned in empty test papers although they had been prepared. They did not want to hurt those friends who were incapable of solving the given tasks.

—Claus Biegert
(*translated by Thomas Poppe*)

If the other person laughs at you, you can pity him;
but if you laugh at him, you may never forgive yourself.
If the other person injures you, you may forget the injury;
but if you injure him, you will always remember.
In truth, the other person is your most sensitive self
   given another body.

—Khalil Gibran, *Sand and Foam*

7

The Center (⓪ and ⑤)

Natural, Vibrant Power

The People of the Center: The Gift of the ⓪ and/or ⑤ in Your Birthdate

Having the gift of the ⓪ or ⑤ in your date of birth assures you stability in almost all life situations. There is very little that will upset the people of the Center. Patience and the willingness to sacrifice, as well as creativity, generosity, and a love of nature, can all be found in the Center. The nurturing care that is at home here creates a strong feeling of rootedness, both in the home environment as well as in sound life principles. The people of the Center exhibit deep spirituality just as often as they do clear reason. In fact, they stand out for their pragmatic thinking and tend to be well liked.

People of the Center like caring unconditionally for someone or something, the helper syndrome is at home in the Numbers of the Center. So, it comes as no surprise that others often take advantage of this helpfulness.

Which way the Center develops on a daily basis strongly depends on the remaining Numbers in the birthdate. This, of course, applies to all Cardinal Points, but in the Center, an additional factor comes into play. The difference between a ⓪ and ⑤ in the date of birth is not particularly dramatic, but it still has a presence. The ⑤ imparts willpower and connectedness to the earth, and is the Number of gardeners and organic farmers. While this mostly holds true for the ⓪ as well, the ⓪ also incorporates a little of all the Numbers and Cardinal Points. Additionally, it has a stronger leaning toward the spiritual aspects of life, making this Number unique. Both the 5 and 0 harbor the energy of the Center, but having the 0 in your birthday gives you a dash of every Number's energy. And although it is in a weaker form than that of the other individual Numbers in your date of birth, the bearers of a 0 and 0 combination tend to have strong personalities. If you want to stay friends with them, you need to let them go on their chosen way.

The Center has an unusual characteristic in that its people frequently suffer from both strong homesickness and strong wanderlust. This is not a contradiction; you have read it correctly. Both extremes are united here, often appearing in the same person. In the words of Goethe's *Faust*, "Two souls reside within my breast." Therefore, creative work that gets one closer to nature can easily accommodate both extremes. These people are often nest builders who do not leave their birthplace or chosen hometown. However, because they feel more intensely and clearly than other people and know that their true roots are not tied to material things or locations, this energy can take on an extreme form, causing them to move frequently.

The patience of the Center can be of great usefulness in various professions, too. Gardeners, organic farmers, foresters, geologists, educators, and others surely have it easier when they begin their path with the 0 or 5. For example, if a person must be physically present all the time at his or her business, having the 0 or 5 in his Code would be of great help.

If you have the Numbers of the Center and have yet to find a profession, or if you do not recognize yourself in what has been said so far, then it might make sense to check out some worldwide philanthropic organizations. This would make it possible to work globally from one central location, potentially fulfilling a lifelong dream.

◆   ◆   ◆   ◆   ◆

Having the Numbers of the Center is comparable to having strong roots. Strangely, in the daily use of language, one characteristic of roots tends to be overlooked. Roots are not only deeply anchored and able to weather all storms but they also enable intense dynamism and movement. They promote the strong growth of the trunk, leaves, and blossoms aboveground. No matter how small and insignificant the root might be, it gives life. Without this germination power, nothing would grow. Although roots never see daylight, they continuously bring life and open the way to the light. This power is immense and lasting. Tiny seeds become huge trees, and flowers break through blacktop.

This integral aspect of growth (or course of actions) through the lure and power of opposite forces makes itself known in the Center through the dangerous futility of any effort. Just as an axe can stop the sap flow of the roots at any time, something similar can happen in life. A tree can sprout anew even after having been deeply wounded. Sometimes, however, the power of the root is not enough; the wounds are too deep. Put in human terms, this metaphor can approximate the helping syndrome of the Center. It is sad and frustrating to lend support and help in vain. But to do so repeatedly in the same situation is a waste of time and energy, and can do damage to the person being helped. It is also an offense against those who would gladly accept your assistance and make good use of it in their day-to-day lives.

One of the main dangers of the Numbers of the Center is being content with the good feeling of helping others or being there for them without paying attention to whether or not this help is effective, genuine, and unconditional. Effective help is always given as assistance to those who are able and willing to help themselves; it is a contribution to the adventure of gaining independence and assuming personal responsibility. True help eventually eliminates its own purpose and moves on to the next task. Dishonest help, on the other hand, robs its object of independence and freedom, and creates material and/or emotional dependence on the helper. This difference is quite apparent in schools. How many teachers nowadays actually express true joy in the progress of their pupils?

Do you observe those qualities in yourself? If so, the antidote has already been found, namely, to be honest with yourself. It works only when you slowly wean yourself of the compulsion that you have to appear good in the eyes of others. This is a big venture, but it is well worth it. At its end beckons true freedom and, above all, the ability to provide true assistance.

Children of the Center

Children of the Center are adventurous; anything can excite them, as long as there is something new to discover. They also like to explore the breadth of what they discover. They want to know all aspects of a matter and are inordinately curious. While all children enjoy a small garden they can take care of, children with a ⓪ or a ⑤ wait for visible success. A child of the Center might say, "I am going to sit here until these seeds sprout." Do not be surprised if they do not give up when there are still no tomatoes days later. It is similar with pet care. A pet, whether it is a dog, turtle, or hamster, will get appropriate care and love for months and years to come. Even after the initial enthusiasm over the new housemate has waned, walking the dog does not become a perfunctory exercise.

To appropriately care for children of the Center, know that all will go well if you encourage their curiosity, their urge to explore, and their love of nature. You may likely contribute to the development of a child who will grow up to help liberate nature and the environment from the mistakes of the twentieth century, and this would be a blessing for the entire world.

Shadows on the Center: The Promise Not Yet Fulfilled

What happens when the successful, pragmatic businessman of the Center reads about the deep closeness to nature in the ⓪ and ⑤ without feeling any solidarity with nature? As with all previous Numbers, we need to look deep and go far back. We need to plunge into our own past. It would be a true waste to not live the ⓪ or ⑤ by rejecting their hidden gifts.

What went wrong here? First of all, we would like to assure you that there is no need to worry if you are at ease with yourself and the world. You have structured your life differently, which is fine. But should you feel that you are not living according to your inner feeling, you might start taking a closer look at the reasons. Perhaps old, wooden, petrified, handed-down values and habits are hampering your life like a ball and chain. For example, many young CEOs go by the old patriarchal, macho culture of their fathers and grandfathers when, in reality, they feel much differently and would rather humanize their companies—with a company day-care program or equal pay for men and women. If, like them, you also feel that you are not living your inner truth, this is your opportunity to do it differently, better. After all, your happiness is what is at stake.

Whatever the reasons behind the deviation from your true self, to uncover your treasure, start with the easiest step. The Center is aligned with the color yellow. Using yellow in your daily life—in your clothing, in your apartment, and at your workplace—will invite the dormant powers of this Station. You will gradually awaken and realize what is available to you again. One thing is certain: whoever has a ⓪ or ⑤ in his or her date of birth should live accordingly, as long as the feeling for it is there.

Initially, it is helpful to saturate and strengthen yourself with these Numbers. For example, choose the ⓪ and ⑤ for daily things like cell phone Numbers, favorite Numbers, license plate Numbers, safe combinations, passwords, and similar things. The ⓪ in the Numbers 10, 20, and so on also count here. What is to stop us from counting 5-10-15-20 instead of 1-2-3? You could do this while cataloging your DVD collection or when numbering the pages of your diary. If someone were to ask you for the reason, tell them. Some people will call this nonsense, but incorporating Numbers into life helps nonetheless.

For men, it is not that simple to include the color yellow in their wardrobe, but a yellow string around their wrist would be sufficient. Our female readers have it easier. Might it be that yellow is already one of your favorite colors? From now on, it will no longer be suppressed but be worn, even in the winter. You know now, of course, what color your new towels might be.

It is not necessary to change careers from being a banker to being a gardener in order to awaken the Center. You may suddenly discover a love for certain plants and grow orchids or cacti. There are many ways to find room for the nature-loving power of the ⓪ and ⑤, even in the smallest city apartment. You could have an herb garden on the windowsill or a mini greenhouse on the balcony.

However, do not forget the following: if you do not recognize yourself in the description of your Cardinal Point and you are totally content with your life, then you have certainly done something in the past that fulfilled the mission of these Numbers. If this is the case, use your imagination to affirm your Center for the continued well-being of all!

When the Center Needs Taming: Development into the Extreme

At first glance, one might assume that the people of the Center rarely experience a damaging, extreme overdevelopment. This is true. However, some people with multiple Units of the ⓪ and ⑤ might find themselves struggling. In everyday life, an overflowing Center might manifest itself in various ways. For example, moderation can escalate to such a degree that it results in a standstill and lethargy. The true moderation of the Center is content with very little but is highly active, mentally and physically. False moderation, on the other hand, is often an external symptom of aimlessness or anxiety.

Do you see yourself as a chronic worrier? Do you allow others to exploit you endlessly until your own feelings and desires fall by the wayside? Absentmindedness and dreaminess are possible signs of an overly strong Center. As is usually the case in life, too much of a good thing turns into the opposite. The dose determines whether it heals or poisons. Generosity taken to the extreme can turn into avarice or extravagance. Wastefulness and dissatisfaction with oneself are an indication that the Center is overdeveloped. Children might display a form of emptiness that cannot be fathomed, or they might be often absentminded.

Here, too, it would be effective to work with colors. Yellow normally enhances creativity and good ideas. However, yellow is not suitable for an overdeveloped Center, which could send you into distraction or a dream world. In this instance, yellow should be mostly avoided, especially when it comes to yellow bed linens and pillowcases. The same holds true for yellow walls and carpets.

As you can see, it is often the small and insignificant things that change the world; all extremes can transition into their opposite. In the case of the 0 and 5, you can no longer speak of the "power of the Center" when you have lost your balance. Therefore, anyone with an overdeveloped Center should generally avoid the color yellow and be more prudent than usual on dates with the 0 and/or 5.

In most cases, it is enough to find a truly fulfilling task. If you are not in a position to make career changes, it is necessary to find a hobby that will compensate. What could be better than the nature lover who gets deeply involved in the computer world, or the extreme internet surfer who finds balance in nature? Spending time around animals also compensates for a strong Center because animals need attention. There is no room for moodiness around them, as they need food and affection even if you have just left your Center again. The more attention you pay, the faster the overdevelopment will find its balance.

When the Center Is Missing: The Birthdate without the 0 and/or 5

If your date of birth contains neither the 0 nor 5 and you do not have the Center in your Wheel, it is not necessary to take a course in organic farming or to go backpacking every Sunday in order to get to know and understand the special powers of the Center. It is enough to meditate for ten minutes every morning in order to stop being blown through life like a leaf in the wind. By the way, earth signs (Taurus, Virgo, and Capricorn) can always fall back on a certain earth-connectedness even if their date of birth does not have a 0 or 5.

We all have days when we feel aimless. Most of the time, this is simply a function of your personal biorhythms (see our book *Moon Time*, page 227) and occurs every fourteen days, starting on the day that you were born. That means you will have one of these days every two weeks on the same day of the week that you were born. It lasts from a few hours to a full day until it is done, and no one can explain its meaning or origin. If the feeling that something is not quite right keeps appearing more and more, it is easy to guess where it is coming from. You are simply lacking the powers of the Center. And fortunately, you do not have to live with that feeling—at least, not as of today. With some rethinking and a little meditation, it is possible to fill this void just by accepting this information. Those who understand causes (versus symptoms alone) have an alternative route to effective medicine.

Let's look briefly at the differences between lacking the **0** and missing the **5**. Without the **5**, there is sometimes a lack of assertiveness in daily life. Without the **0**, the inner Center is missing. As a result, it is rare that a person feels entirely satisfied with themselves; there is a persistent urge to check if everything is done well enough, even if the success is already obvious. We feel a certain emptiness and ask ourselves if we have done, chosen, or achieved the right things in life. A child without the Center sometimes suffers from anxiety and may need something nest-like at home, such as a pile of stuffed animals or other comforting items, to create a substitute for the missing sense of belonging.

Successful counterbalance is important here. On days without scheduled plans or on a special occasion, simply make sure that the feeling of emptiness passes quickly or does not have a chance to surface in the first place. One highly effective solution is to cultivate a closeness to nature. However, this cannot always be done spontaneously. Therefore, we have another trick available for acute cases: have contact with animals. For children, a pet can be extremely helpful. It can be small, too, like a hamster or a guinea pig. Or when choosing a destination for a day trip, consider a farm or a petting zoo. Even a neighbor's dog or cat can help.

Children who do not have the Center enjoy having their own little garden. Allow them to have the adventure of planting things themselves and of observing nature—of sowing flower seeds, and of following small animals and insects in their garden. For these children, it is extremely beneficial to participate in the natural rhythm of growing, ripening, and harvesting—the ending and the new beginning.

Adults can strengthen their Center by choosing reading materials that help to focus and ground them. Frequently, day-to-day life catches up with us, leaving us too little time to find our Center. It is highly useful to pay attention to energy-robbing tendencies in order to enjoy the time for other things. Make and keep a schedule, as it is much more enjoyable to indulge in daydreaming when you know ahead of time that you are not going to wake up with a bad conscience.

Let us return to the colors once more. When in doubt, pick yellow. Since yellow is the color you are lacking, it is the color that can awaken your Center. Using it as your dominant color is a simple daily exercise that will help you to slowly get closer to the missing Center. For example, you can paint entire walls yellow or decorate using the "power of sunflowers." Yellow curtains are visible even when open, and they can make a house very livable. You could also set up a yellow "snuggle corner," even if you are already an adult. There is no age limit for what is right, good, and healthy!

Medicine for the Soul

Anybody can sympathize with the sufferings of a friend,
But it requires a very fine nature to sympathize with
a friend's success.

—Oscar Wilde

We need not continue living
As we lived yesterday.
Free yourself from this perception,
And a thousand possibilities invite us to a new life.

—Christian Morgenstern
(**translated by Thomas Poppe**)

You ask yourself why it is so important,
Why all great teachers preach

That we should feel thankful?
There are many reasons
That you can only find out personally,
But we can name one of the most important ones:
No one can be thankful and
Feel unhappy at the same time.

—**Ron Fischer**

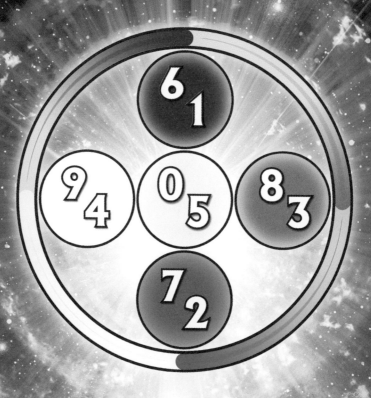

Part 3

The Signatures

Introduction to the Signatures

The Number Wheel has exactly thirty-one possible combinations of Cardinal Points that can arise from birthday Numbers. We refer to these thirty-one unique combinations as the Signatures. To begin, we would like to familiarize you with this colorful arrangement of Numbers and colors that make up the Signatures, as well as with your very own bouquet.

In order to understand the Code, the first and most important step is for you to read about your Cardinal Points in part 2. This is where you can read about what is in your personal treasure chest. After that, there are essentially two possibilities. First, you may discover that you already have intuitively made the best of your Numbers' bounty. Wonderful! Congratulations! Alternately, in the second scenario, you might discover that you do not recognize yourself in the description. People often tell us, "I have always felt what you are telling me about myself. But, you know, I never fully developed that part of myself because of circumstances at the time / my parents / my teachers / my bosses," and so on.

It is by no means our intention to urge you to turn your life upside down. But you must no longer moan over missed opportunities either. Complaining might work at your local bar, with friends at a coffee shop, in a law office, or during therapy. However, complaining costs energy, and it achieves nothing worthwhile. You will only get on the last nerves of those who are already on their way to making the best of their lives. You, too, should be on your way. The Birthday Wheel and your personal Signature are your guideposts. From now on, you will have the tools you need to manage your own life.

Everyone, of course, has a different story to tell about how they got their start in life. Your personal soul-building process determines your challenges, whether you are too shy, too scared, too naive, too reproachful, too distrustful, too stingy, too weak, too greedy, too lazy, too tired, or too sick.

Whatever gets you down in life, put an end to it! Concentrate on your many positive qualities from now on, and make the best of them. If certain situations make you feel too apprehensive, or too this or that, the feeling in itself is not bad. But beware when this temporary way of thinking (and it is only that) becomes a pillar of your day-to-day life. When you find yourself saying, "I know what is right, but I cannot do it differently," take a look at the wonderful qualities conferred from your Cardinal Points in part 2. You already have your Number treasure; start making something good from it now.

Everything becomes easier with the correct tools. A watchmaker needs different instruments than an organic baker, and an Indy race car driver needs a different machine than a farmer in the field. Neither trade is better or worse than the other. The farmer cannot use a race car to bring in the harvest, nor can the race-car driver win a flowerpot trophy with a tractor. The watchmaker cannot use a precision screwdriver to bake rolls, just as the organic baker cannot use a wooden spoon to repair watches. It is that simple.

Use your talents to reach your goal, whatever it may be. There should be room for all people on this planet, because we need everyone. Look without recrimination at your weaknesses, negative tendencies, and habits. Do it tomorrow, then do it again the next day. And after some time passes, do it once again. In some things, we do not know ourselves as well as an outsider does. Taking an honest look at ourselves in the mirror is not an easy task; every person has a shadow side. The basic law, however, says that the more honest we are with ourselves, the faster we will find our personal path toward light, happiness, and a love for life.

If a child lives with fairness, he learns justice.
If a child lives with criticism, he learns to condemn.
If a child lives with security, he learns to have faith.
If a child lives with hostility, he learns to fight.
If a child lives with approval, he learns to like himself.
If a child lives with shame, he learns to feel guilty.
If a child lives with encouragement, he learns confidence.
If a child lives with ridicule, he learns to be shy.
If a child lives with tolerance, he learns to be patient.
If a child lives with acceptance and friendship,
*   he learns to find love in the world.*

Author Unknown
(**Sign at Guthrie Castle, Scotland**)

8. The Five Singles

The North

Genius and the open door to the world–
all powers point upward

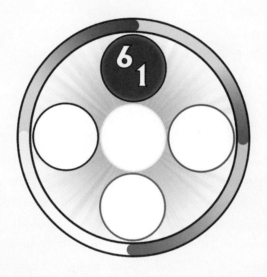

Wisdom and love have been building the world since eternity
And create spring meadows from night and winter time;
Their magic rules everywhere, rejuvenating the old
And forcing out the cold with a fiery word!

—Hermann Lingg
(translated by Thomas Poppe)

This Signature contains dates of birth with the Numbers

❻ and/or ❶

The birthdates January 6, 1961; June 1, 1916; January 1, 1966; and June 6, 1911, are all examples of the North Signature—a very rare combination.

If you have read this book from the beginning, you might be curious (and maybe a little anxious as well) about what it may mean that only one of your Stations in the Birthday Wheel is occupied. Do not worry; all Signatures lead to success in life. You merely need to know how to uncover the treasure in your Code—to plainly and simply be the genius that you are.

Having only the ❻ or ❶ in one's Signature indicates above-average intelligence. We are not referring to scientific reasoning and logic, which is like a reliable vehicle that can take you anywhere, but rather to the intelligence—the instinct—that turns life into a meaningful journey. There is no way of predicting which direction the genius of this Signature will take. One might become an extraordinary politician, a true servant of the state. Another might become the best carpenter in the country. Whatever this person does, he or she will want—and deserve—to be heard. Among many with this Signature, you will find top journalists with abilities that others only dream about, and courage that changes the world.

If someone with this Signature is born into a family with the motto "Where would we be if everyone behaved like you?" then this person of the pure North has the likely potential to become insecure. Despite all of his or her talents, this person might gradually become convinced that he or she is mentally inadequate. People with this Signature can only maintain and nurture their genius if they are influenced by people who understand and encourage them. This can come from a distant relative, a special teacher who can look beneath the surface of her students and love them, or even a friend at the gym. You have the power to consciously summon such growth-enhancing influences. Everyone can be a good gardener to the delicate plant of the soul at any time.

The true genius of this Signature must be turned into something fruitful for the self or for the world, or its bearer will soon be considered an oddball or outsider. A difficult child can turn into a directionless adult who can find neither the right career nor the right friends. In daily life, this person is often clumsy and cannot even find matching socks in the morning. (Especially brilliant people tend to fail in the routines of day-to-day life.) All they need, however, is the encouragement and smart teamwork inspired by one or several colleagues. With it, a person of the North can think through, usher in, and market a brilliant product or idea successfully. It is here where the good can lie fallow. The implementation and marketing tasks simply need to be handled by others. Everything should be organized and secured contractually from all sides.

Additionally, this Signature can encounter emotional problems because insight and the ability to see the big picture are lacking. The appropriate colors and the right food could awaken the missing complementary energies and make them accessible; even the simplest measures produce a resounding effect. First, do away with the colors black and blue in your clothing and environment—you have enough of them. Increased use of these colors might awaken or amplify the tendency to go to extremes. Choose green when emotions are involved, red if you need increased vitality, yellow to search for peace and ideas, and white when you need to take care of business. Skillfully choosing color combinations will allow you to better manage everyday life.

Small, appropriately colored scarves offer one way of dappling in color without going to extremes. You can wear them inconspicuously, or you can use them to make your wardrobe more colorful. The latter, of course, depends on your chosen profession and gender. Unusual color combinations are not tolerated in every environment, even if their purpose is to complete your inner self.

When it comes to selecting your food, pay careful attention to color. It might take a while before the scientific community comprehends what every child knows instinctively, but we can tell you here and now that the actual color of food has a health value unto its own that is independent of its verifiable ingredients. Someone who eats mostly pale-colored food like rice, potatoes, and pasta will also develop a pallid personality. Look at the rainbow-colored variety found on the dinner table in Mediterranean countries. Choose multicolored or white plates and cups (or at least colored table linens and/or napkins) when you are preparing your table.

Further, as person of the North, you might prefer something simple like carrying a healing Number. In that case, just write all your missing Numbers on a small piece of paper and carry it on your person at all times. We understand that this advice might sound outlandish, but do it anyway—surreptitiously if necessary. It takes very little effort, and it works. You do not need to know more.

Genius and failure are only separated by a fine line. If you are not satisfied with your life, start over as of today. Perhaps you need a different occupation. Take a look around to see who or what slows you down or lifts you up; you have the right to choose all who bring you happiness. Surround yourself with people who accept you. You should definitely go back to part 2 and read the paragraph about the Numbers of the North—the ❻ and ❶ (starting on page 25). They are your treasure chest full of riches! There, you will find ideas for career and life choices that would make the best of your abilities. Devote yourself also to reading the chapters about your missing Stations to better understand areas that need to be balanced. This is the path to contentment and happiness.

The East

Deep empathy, musicality, and the gift to heal—
all in intense, concentrated form

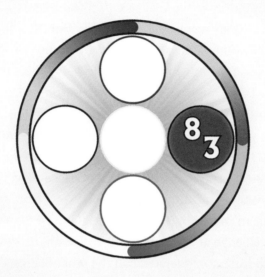

Our bodies are our gardens, to the which
our wills are gardeners: so that if we will plant nettles,
or sow lettuce, set hyssop, and weed up thyme,
supply it with one gender of herbs, or distract it with many,
either to have it sterile with idleness,
or manured with industry,
why, the power and corrigible authority of this
lies in our wills.

—William Shakespeare, *Othello*

This Signature contains dates of birth with the Numbers

8 and/or 3

The birthdates March 8, 1983: August 3, 1933; March 3, 1938; and August 8, 1988, are all examples of the very rare East Signature.

This Signature represents the East in its purest form with its one-of-a-kind qualities—musicality, empathy, the ability to heal, and more. Good-naturedness, fairness, and readiness to help others are highly developed here as well. Do you have this rare Signature? If so, it is probably not easy for you to fully actualize those qualities on a day-to-day basis. This is mainly because you cannot understand why others do not have as much empathy as you have. Some people with this Signature have the constant feeling that all surfaces in their surroundings are covered with thorns. For them, every movement hurts.

Though it is an incredibly valuable gift, the East Signature represents an enormous challenge at the same time. If you are its bearer, it is one of your life tasks to learn to understand all the other Stations of the Birthday Wheel. At first, you might find the temperamental, fiery way of the South a little stressful and the balancing, earthy energy of the Center too boring and bland. As a stranger to the stubborn power of the West, you may initially perceive it as being quite ruthless, and the intense energies of the North might frighten you. You may feel closest to the intuitive quality of the Center. Understanding each, however, will allow you to conquer each territory and gain sovereignty over your entire Birthday Wheel. All in all, beautiful challenges lie ahead of you in life.

A strong East often brings with it great tolerance—a general "live and let live" attitude—since nothing in human behavior is strange to the people of the East. For this reason, the Signature of the East is known to have a calming effect on others, and its bearers slowly earn the role of being the first people everyone consults; it is a safe harbor against the many storms in the world. And this is right in line with the nature of the East, which derives great pleasure from feeling needed.

If you are a bearer of this Signature, your home and heart are wide open to an abundance of influences. The word "no" is a skill among your emotional equipment that must be painstakingly learned. It is common to find yourself in situations where you agree without meaning to, though you may be saying no in your own language. You may briefly shake your head, for example, or turn it to avoid eye contact. Or you might breathe faster or say, "Yes, but…," and naturally, the other person will only hear "yes." You may know ten thousand ways to say no, but your indirect manner leaves the back door open for the other person to hear yes.

Stop hoping that your subtle signals will be understood, and learn to say no honestly and directly. If you don't, both you and the people around you will suffer because you might have to get angry before others understand your true wishes. But it never has to get to this point. Avoid this shocking extreme by relying on the other tools in your chest—your patience and highly tuned sense of nuance. Learn to speak your desires the same way.

The need to help is rooted in your Signature, but where and when should your natural helpfulness flow? The answer to that usually requires inspiration and encouragement from outside help. In your eyes, the organizational aspects surrounding the activity of helping are for the most part superfluous and unnecessarily delay things. Rightfully so! Helping comes first; bureaucracy can wait.

In order to counteract the constant exploitation of your best qualities, you need to make a conscious effort to conquer your missing Stations. An effective, immediate measure would be to wisely add in some colors. The vibrancy of the missing South (❼/❷) is best integrated into your life by using the color red. The empty West (❾/❹) awaits the wise application of the color white (clothing works well). White will ensure that people become more aware of you as it also helps you to develop the energies and qualities of the West—determination, precision, and organizational skills. Prevent the shortchanging of the North by generously using the colors black and blue, and attract the earthy, balancing energies of the Center (❶/5) with yellow. Choosing the right colors can influence many things quickly and effectively.

People with few Stations occupied in their Signature sometimes instinctively compensate for the voids by decorating their environment or adding color to their wardrobe. Perhaps you know people with only one Station in their Signatures whose homes are intensely hued with multi-colored cushions, rainbows on the walls, and other colorful details, using throw rugs and knickknacks to cover virtually every inch of their home. When friends with more than one Cardinal Point come to visit, this type of environment can overwhelm or confuse them, or put them in a downcast mood without apparent reason. However, you should trust your intuition and treat yourself to this permanent array of colors within your four walls.

You can also colorfully decorate your workplace by using colored quartz. Green is the only color that should be used sparingly, as you have inherited enough of that color. You can find out which professions would make you happy by reading the paragraph about the Numbers of the East in part 2 (starting on page 41). You will find suggestions there for the general direction you are meant to take. If your current profession does not make you happy, make a change! It is never too late. If this is not possible, devote your free time to your talents. Every moment that you spend doing something that makes you happy is worth it!

The South

Fiery temperament, enthusiasm, and charisma—
all under one roof

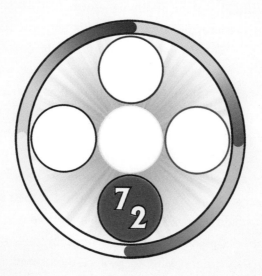

It is so pleasant to explore Nature and oneself
at the same time,
doing violence neither to her nor to one's own spirit,
But bringing both into balance
In gentle, mutual interaction.

—Johann Wolfgang von Goethe

This Signature contains dates of birth with the Numbers

7 and/or 2

The birthdates July 27, 1972; February 2, 1977; July 2, 1927; and February 7, 1922, are all examples of the South Signature.

Just like the two previous Signatures, this Signature also describes a very unique person. The person of the South is full of vitality. If a person with this Signature becomes an actress or actor, no bell will be needed to quiet the audience to get them to listen. This will happen solely because of this person's charismatic presence.

Such people are not overlooked and are extremely resentful if someone dares to try. A heavy 7 and 2 Signature belongs in the public eye, as its bearers generate enthusiasm and sweep people off their feet. Drab office buildings and gray surroundings are not their world or their stage; their energies and abilities would be wasted in such an environment.

People of the South have little talent for being hermits. In extreme situations, however, they might want to protect themselves from their own temperament and may yearn for the life of a monk. But this rarely happens; the South's inner happiness lies on the outside. They need contact with other people and do best in ventures that do not require a long start-up period. They make a plan and implement it immediately, getting straight to the point without taking detours! These are the people of the South.

Naturally, impatience is not foreign to a person with this Signature, who shows little tolerance for a long wait at the dentist or drive-up window— or stoppages of any kind. A pure person of the South can handle many situations efficiently but finds the detailed organization and preparation too time-consuming. They are, therefore, no strangers to temper tantrums (which are almost second nature), and they are always puzzled by the astonished and frightened faces around them afterward.

Children with this Signature are told in no uncertain terms—and more often than others—to quiet down. The stronger and more frequent the reprimands, the greater the likelihood that such a child will sink into resignation and lose direction. Though externally peaceful, this child will be a volcano inside, waiting to explode.

Suppressed feelings lead to physical symptoms, and as a person with this Signature, you will most likely suffer more frequently from fevers (also an external sign of a weakened immune system). You can effectively counteract this with cold compresses, blue clothing, and blue bed linens.

If any of this sounds familiar to you, it is even more important to start the quest of conquering the remaining Stations of the Birthday Wheel. Just resist the temptation to conquer everything with brute strength and gritted teeth. Patiently allow your understanding to grow instead.

Consider taking the time now to leisurely reacquaint yourself with your missing Stations—West (**9**/**4**), North (**6**/**1**), East (**8**/**3**), and Center (**0**/ **5**)—by reading the corresponding sections in part 2. At first glance, this might seem like a lot of material, but your life adventure is not a weekend trip! Look at it this way: by having such a pure Signature, you have a lot of genius to offer in your field. All you have to do is to awaken the life in the missing Numbers. And remember that you need not bother with the negative energies that are inevitably present on the shadow side of those Signatures. Just focus on the positive.

Over time, you will feel the compensation for the missing Stations. Experience shows that the wise use of colors is an effective immediate measure. It is best to attend to a strong South by using the color red sparingly, in clothing as well as in the colors of your home or workplace.

The missing West (**9**/**4**), on the other hand, awaits the wise use of the color white (best used in clothing). With its special energy of the West, white ensures that you develop willpower, precision, and organizational skills, which complement the fiery impetuousness of your Signature.

Green is the color of the East (**8**/**3**) and a source for more patience and sensibility on an emotional level. Walking more often in nature is good compensation for the innate impatience of your Signature.

The color yellow summons the special earthy and balancing energies of the Center (**0**/**5**), and smooths the way to levelheadedness and a sense of proportion.

Maximize the curious, searching, idea-rich North (**❻**/**❶**) by using black and/or blue generously. You can also obtain its healing, balancing energy by working with partners whose Signatures contain the North Station.

Each Signature has its own characteristics and weaknesses, and in your case, developing the ability to be part of a team would be a big step forward. The abilities needed for that will help you conquer the missing Stations of your Birthday Wheel. We wish you much luck!

The West

Destined to succeed–
a talent thankfully accepted

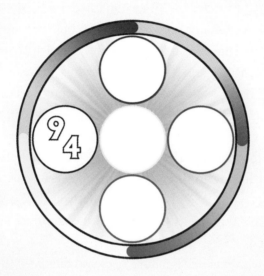

Do you think you can take over the universe and improve it?
I do not believe it can be done.
The universe is sacred.
You cannot improve it.
If you try to change it, you will ruin it.
If you try to hold it, you will lose it.

So sometimes things are ahead and sometimes they are behind;
Sometimes breathing is hard, sometimes it comes easily;
Sometimes there is strength and sometimes weakness;
Sometimes one is up and sometimes down.
Therefore the sage avoids extremes, excesses, and complacency.
—Lao Tzu

This Signature contains dates of birth with the Numbers

9 and/or **4**

The birthdates April 4, 1949; April 9, 1944; September 4, 1994; September 9, 1949; and April 4, 1994, are all examples of the West Signature. These Numbers are connected not only to the West, but they are also extremely rare. The next opportunity will not come until April 4, 2044.

This **9**/**4** Signature and its energies need to be treated very carefully and consciously. An above-average talent for running a business, a strictly success-based orientation, and a high intelligence are all present in this Signature. And since you only have one Station occupied, a lot of Units bunch up here to provide additional fuel for your strengths. This creates the challenge of having to direct all of this powerful energy of the West into meaningful channels. One might say that you have a very strong and fast horse available that needs to be taught the appropriate boundaries in order to be tamed.

Everything within your Signature rises and falls with the right proportions and the wise application of energies. Many people around you end up feeling overwhelmed, which might result in a problem: people may feel they cannot measure up to you at times, no matter how good they are or how hard they try. You may not be aware of it, but danger lurks in the form of a general resignation that spreads through those around you. Very few people have your talents, so one of your tests is to understand when others are not as business savvy as you. Even though your genius intuits an easily recognizable, sensible direction, this skill is the exception and not the rule.

Here is a little hint about your happiness in this lifetime. Do not expect to be totally understood—ever. Your speed of doing things is a tough act to follow, and you bring such goal orientation to your life path that it leaves little room for abilities that you do not understand or appreciate.

Here, we would like to call out to you, "Not for long." Despite all the success you might have earned based upon your special talents, your key to true happiness in life lies in broadening your horizons to include the inherent qualities and talents of the other Stations of the Number Wheel. For example, your manual skills might be legendary but might also turn you into a loner. After all, you do not need anyone; no one can do it better than you. Teamwork is not your cup of tea because you feel it squanders time. You also frequently feel that it stifles your energies.

You need to study the elixir of music or the life-giving energies of a garden. Live your genius, but in the future, leave a little more room for things not yet present. Try to develop the understanding that other people whose abilities are not as strong as yours are merely distributing their treasure differently; their abilities just have different forms and colors. Of course, if you measure success by the size of your bank account, the creation of a company day-care center or your daughter's music recital become secondary. Look! Here is your key: a tree might be loaded with fruit, but without roots, branches, leaves, bees, the rays of the sun, and many other elements, there would have been none.

Since your Signature is missing four Stations of the Birthday Wheel, it could be that you do not feel totally content, despite your achievements and recognition, or you feel that your contentment is gradually fading away. You are not alone in this, but no one can teach you how to be truly happy—not teachers, schools, parents, religion, therapists, or any other helping professions or institutions. Where could we possibly learn this lesson anyway? Although we do not have to move an inch, for most of us, this is the longest journey of them all. If peace and self-love are missing, you do not have the insight you need to look into your heart. Every trip around the world starts with one single step, however, and your journey to happiness is no exception.

As always, you can acquire the abilities of the missing Stations with the help of the appropriate colors. Avoid wearing white as much as possible, even though professions of the West are often held by one of your people wearing white! White is the color of the West, and you have more than enough of its charisma. Do not select a workspace that faces the West or is situated in the West part of a building, whether at home or work. You should also avoid vacation spots oriented to the West. To provide balance, the first choice should be the East. Second would be the South and the North. It would also be sensible to live in a geographic Center—near the town square, in a city center, or downtown, for example.

Do not forget to integrate the healing power of color in your life. Your Signature benefits most from green—in your clothing, your household, your food, and so on. However, blue, black, yellow, and red also help. Orange (the combination of red and yellow) has a soothing effect as well. For your food, "multicolored" is the word. You should never eat colorless or pale foods over a long period of time. This includes pasta, rice, potatoes, white sauces, pound cakes with sugar icing, and so on.

With the exception of the ❾ and ❹, all Numbers can complement and balance your Signature. Avoid the ❾ and ❹ whenever possible—on license plates, house Numbers, room Numbers in hotels, and above all, in telephone Numbers. Time to read part 2 again (starting on page 29) to understand the meaning of the missing Stations. If you manage to spend a day once in a while "just hanging out" with your friends, you will have accomplished much toward wholeness and true happiness.

The Center

The patient wanderer between two worlds—
at home in the inner and the outer world

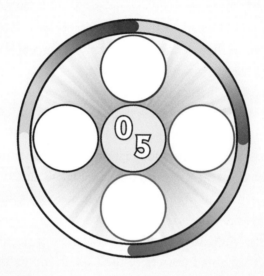

If we are connected like brothers by a common goal outside of us,
only then will we breathe freely and learn that Love is not just looking at each other,
But it is looking together in the same direction.
Comrades are those who unite on the same rope and climb—
the same mountain summit to find themselves.
Why are we so deeply happy, in this age of comfort,
to share our last food with each other in the desert?

—Antoine de Saint-Exupéry
(*translated by Thomas Poppe*)

This Signature contains dates of birth with the Numbers

⓪ and/or ⑤

The birthdates May 5, 1900; May 5, 1905; May 5, 1950; May 5, 1955; May 5, 2000; and May 5, 2005, are all examples of the Center Signature. In addition to being connected to the Signature of the Center, they are the only dates of birth in the twentieth and twenty-first centuries that contain the Numbers of the Center until May 5, 2050.

People with this Signature are specially equipped to deal with extreme situations, and they will encounter a number of them in life. However, the powers of the Center (⓪/⑤) carry a comforting attribute: this Signature does not feel the severity of such extreme situations—mainly because the power of the Center grants quick access to solutions. Difficult situations barely have time to make a permanent impression on your memory. One person's catastrophe is this Signature's hiccup.

Of course, this Signature also has its own set of peculiar battles and foes. The heavily weighted powers of the Center and its large number of challenges sometimes assail this Signature in quick succession and carry a hidden danger. The people with this Signature occasionally experience feelings of crippling resignation followed by a sigh and the thought, "Not again!" It may feel like too much to have to gather oneself and take action once again. At those moments, we need to remember with deep conviction that our Guiding Spirit won't give us more to bear than we can handle.

Interestingly, two extremes meet within the Signature of the Center—rooted domesticity and seemingly restless wandering. Having a Number twice in the Center (⓪ or ⑤) is sometimes enough to put down roots in the same place for the rest of one's life or to move from place to place, maybe even in a camper. It could also happen that one divides life into phases, not moving for twenty years and then uprooting and spending the next year in many different towns, never fully unpacking the suitcases. As you found out in part 2, the power of the Center is the power that encompasses all Cardinal Points and also radiates out to them. When you have the Center in your date of birth, conquering all other Stations and their specific qualities is not that big a challenge. Perhaps this makes it easier to understand this inner conflict.

Both extremes, domesticity and wanderlust, might join in one person and change constantly. For example, as a child, you may have *always* wanted to get away, but as a young adult, you *always* stay home. Suddenly, in middle age, everything turns around; the life of a vagabond beckons (and is often chosen). If you feel or have felt this wavering back and forth, you now know that it is a part of the typical nature of the Center.

As a person of the Center, your empathy toward people and situations tends to fluctuate wildly between high sensitivity and cool indifference, though the latter happens rarely. Generally, the bearers of this Signature are understanding people who can take on greatly varying roles, and they stand out in their forbearance. You often find the energy of the ⓪ and ⑤ represented in professions that require endless patience and dedication. Of course, the energy of the "other side"—the dark side where rage lives— hovers in the air. As you probably gathered from reading about the preceding Signatures, the power of the Center is in concentrated form, however, and concentrated Units in any one direction, including the Center, carry with them the danger of unexplained actions, sudden outbursts of temper, and so on. In this case, the unexpected should not surprise you.

We already indicated that the special quality of a Signature of the Center with the ⓪ is its ability to feel the energies and qualities of the other Numbers. This means that this Signature unites all the gifts of the Birthday Wheel or has easy access if so desired—unless, of course, it was unlearned or affected by fear during one's childhood.

When it comes to color for the Center Signature, you should definitely avoid the color yellow in your clothing, at the workplace, and at home. Dare to wear and surround yourself with many colors.

If a Signature's Center of Gravity is located in the Center, especially with this Signature, it would be wise to meditate. As mentioned earlier, the dark "other side" of insight and patience is rage, and unprocessed and unresolved rage takes a toll on your inner organs.

The body's detoxifying organs—liver, kidneys, pancreas, lymph nodes, spleen, stomach, and intestines—require more attention and care with this Signature. A good preventive measure is to drink a purifying tea (such as nettle) during a waning moon between 3 PM and 7 PM. During a waning moon, you should also be more careful about what you eat.

Despite the seeming one-sidedness of your Numbers, you have everything you need in the Center Signature to make a happy life for yourself and those around you. Just take good care of yourself and the rest will follow.

9. The Ten Doubles

North–East

Keen intuition and a sharp look behind the scenes—
the big picture beckons

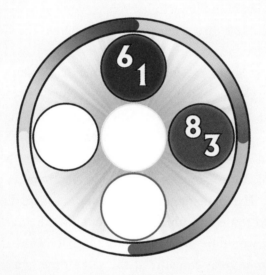

If you want to be loved, start loving others who need your love.
If you want others to sympathize with you,
start showing sympathy to those around you.
If you want to be respected, you must learn to be respectful to everyone,
both young and old.
Whatever you want others to be, first be that yourself;
then you will find others responding in like manner to you.

—**Paramahansa Yogananda**

This Signature contains dates of birth with the Numbers

6 and/or **1**
8 and/or **3**

The birthdates March 16, 1968; June 13, 1986; August 6, 1938; March 13, 1986; and June 1, 1913, are all examples of the North–East Signature. There are, of course, many additional combinations possible.

When working with the Birthday Wheel, you need to carefully observe which Numbers make up a given Signature. Where is the Center of Gravity located? The two dates of birth, August 1, 1988, and June 3, 1966, have the same North–East Signature, for example, but the Center of the first is in the East and the Center of the second is in the North. Aside from environmental and hereditary variations, a different treasure chest is available in each birthdate, and two different characters will form. The Centers of Gravity within a Signature have more significance when there are only two Stations available for the four to six possible Numbers, as is the case with the North–East. The Signature provides an approximate direction.

If we were to come up with a clever catchphrase for each Signature, the best choice here would be "intelligent intuition." Recognizing deep interrelations and having great empathy at the same time is a rare gift. In this Signature, this gift comes to life. However, it might first need awakening in some who bear it. Both abilities are like tender young plants; when they lack adequate care, they have trouble sprouting. But they do exist and are waiting to come into their own!

People with this Signature find learning easy. They understand things quickly and remember them for a long time. The prerequisite is that they are interested in the given subject. If that is not the case, parents and teachers sometimes find them a hard nut to crack and may resort to tutoring as a way to awaken their sleeping curiosity. In general, however, children with this Signature do not need help with their homework.

When a Signature combines the North and the East, if offers a large variety of fascinating fields. Nature and world events are the main directions of interest. The North stands for intelligence and intellect; the East represents intuition and perseverance in musicality and healing.

This Signature has only one big disadvantage: at times, one might take too long to understand a situation and end up acting upon it too late. Also, the energy of the North (❻/❶) can provoke extreme impatience when its bearers do not receive support or appreciation for their flights of fancy. This will make them more likely to resign. And, putting it bluntly, the East is the home of self-pity when things do not go according to plans, desires, or dreams. (Self-pity ranks high on the list of time wasters.) It would be best to pull the emergency brake on self-love and self-responsibility when you feel a wave of resignation coming.

The bearers of this Signature generally manage well in life because they have learned that they do not have to master everything themselves. Successful Signature holders in general should, whenever possible, pass on their talents to others for the sake of fulfilling one's purpose. In the best-case scenario, these are passed to the next Station in the rotation of the Birthday Wheel—to the South in this instance (see page 13). Give your special talents not only to your partner and counterpart in business life but also privately to those who display the South, West, and Center in the Wheel. The assistance of these partners and friends is beneficial in implementing a wide variety of plans.

Every Signature has challenges to overcome; in your case, it is gullibility. For example, partners who are blessed with many ❾s and ❹s are sometimes prone to grab well-earned success from people who have a missing West. You can be careless, too generous, and too naive in financial dealings. People do not necessarily take advantage with evil intentions, but they may grab an opportunity if the North–East Signature makes it too easy for them. They might even believe that the exploitation is fine, saying, "I really did not mean anything by it and would have paid everything back eventually."

Having an empty South can result in a lack of self-confidence at times, even when there is no actual reason. For example, when a Nobel Prize–winner lacks the ❼ or ❷ in his or her birthdate, this person might ask inwardly at times if the prize was truly earned. The missing West (❾/❹) creates a void that is felt in business situations—the "fire in the belly" disappears when it is most needed. A missing Center (0 / 5) is of relatively little consequence here because the East heavily populates the world of emotions, creating equilibrium.

Should you be a person of this Signature and see yourself more as an insecure person, then you should work with a lot of red in your life—in your clothing as well as your home and workplace. It would be invigorating for you to frequently have red fruit, berries, and vegetables on the menu. Or wear something crazy! Let's assume you feel that you do not get attention in public next to your friends or partner. At the next public outing or social gathering, wear bright red instead of black and enjoy the attention you get as you outdo your partner. The only prerequisite is that you feel comfortable doing this and do not just do it to be noticed. Otherwise, it is merely embarrassing and moves you no closer to conquering the Code. Use white for business meetings to strengthen your willpower and assertiveness. At home, yellow should prevail over green, black, and blue. Your Signature has enough of those colors.

Equipped with insight in the inner dynamics of your Signature, you are off to a good start.

East–South

Cheerful, helpful, and empathetic— very lively if taken care of properly

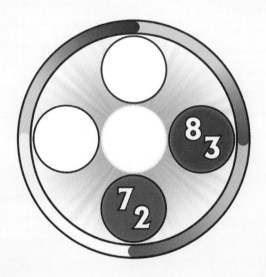

Truth is like the stars;
it does not appear except from behind obscurity of the night.
Truth is like all beautiful things in the world;
it does not disclose its desirability except to those who first feel the influence of falsehood.
Truth is a deep kindness that teaches us to be content in our everyday life
and share with the people the same happiness.

—Khalil Gibran

This Signature contains dates of birth with the Numbers

8 and/or **3**
7 and/or **2**

The birthdates August 3, 1972; July 2, 1978; February 8, 1938; July 27, 1987; and August 7, 1927, are all examples of the East–South Signature. However, these dates represent only a few examples for this combination of Cardinal Points.

A special life adventure awaits the bearer of this Signature. Peace-loving and nature-connected sensitivity is paired with a sense of freedom and vibrancy, but these energies need to be tamed and united under one roof. If this is successful, a fulfilled life beckons. When we meet people with this Signature, they are frequently cheerful and likeable, and are welcome everywhere. They have a healthy measure of self-confidence but know when enough is enough. You rarely find boring types in the East–South who tell endless jokes. This is why bearers of this Signature tend to be favorite party guests. They help create a good atmosphere for a pleasant get-together, and you can almost bet that they are the ones who will stay and help clean-up afterward. They even made a positive impression as children when invited to birthday parties. We would miss this Signature, were it not to exist.

Altogether, this Signature has many permutations, and a colorful life awaits. The balance of the compass points can swing strongly toward the East or the South, or it can remain fairly equal. The fiery temperament of the South will become more prominent when the East has only one **8** or one **3**. Conversely, the soul will feel calmer if the South contains a single **2** (August 2, 1983, for example). It is then that the emotions move to the forefront, and the Southern temperament cools down.

The bearers of this Signature tend to be musical. You will often find a musical instrument in his or her closet that is not a dust collector but a much-played specimen that contributes to the good mood of the user and listeners alike. People of this Signature need not be encouraged to sing either; they enjoy it as much as we enjoy listening. As physicians, alternative healers, traditional healers, or veterinarians, they prefer working with their intuition. The missing Center is of lesser importance here, since the thoughtfulness of the East compensates for a great deal. The empty West (❾/❹), however, leaves a definite void that should be actively balanced in later years. Business matters, part of the domain of the West, need to be kept under control. Good physicians—those who are true friends of humanity, who became physicians to heal and not for financial reward—would do well wearing white all the time. White is the color of the West, representing willpower and the ability to strike a balance between give and take. People with an East–South Signature can compensate for their initial lack of business sense by teaming up with competent partners. They might also make a conscious decision to learn what would fill their particular voids of knowledge and understanding by reading this book in its entirety.

The missing West (❾/❹) prevents people with this Signature from implementing their good ideas and improvements. A professional partner with the West in his or her date of birth could provide the additional energy an East–South bearer needs and could work in such a way that both benefit from the relationship.

It is interesting that the best physicians in the world often have this Signature, even though they have not studied a long time. Academia is not for them, as they do not have the endurance of the North—a virtual prerequisite for lengthy studies. It would be beneficial for those in this Signature to persevere with their studies if they intend to become physicians or alternative healers. Such physicians would have the ability to actually help patients address the true causes of their illnesses.

The dislike of studying also applies to musicians. When the North (❻/❶) is empty, a person is not inclined to spend a long time in school. This is not a reflection on ability; it merely indicates that the will is not there. If someone has decided to walk a path of academic learning and all of the work it entails, the energies of the East and the South are surely enough to be successful. But why make life difficult? Use the colors of your intuitive

Center (yellow) and the wise North (black or blue) along the way. Black helps us to turn inward and meditate until our unfailing inner voice becomes audible. Yellow provides new ideas and inspiration. Use these colors in your clothing, your home, and your workplace, or use them as small pieces of paper that you can carry around with you. Little by little, you will begin to feel a change in your mood.

It would not be advisable to use red bed linens for a child with this Signature. Red linens could result in restless sleep since the South is already present in the child. When a mother herself does not have the **❼** or **❷** in her date of birth, she could mistakenly feel that red would benefit her East–South child. However, white or yellow would be the ideal color choices in this case. This also holds true for adults, who can do their own shopping (children often have to settle for what they get). The missing Center (**0**/**5**) has a lesser impact in this instance since the East provides emotional balance. However, if you feel the lack yourself, long walks in nature and the use of yellow in your daily life will help to fill the void.

Altogether, this is a very lively Signature whose talents are many. Give this gift to yourself and the world.

South–West

With vigor and ambition toward your goal–
on a good path

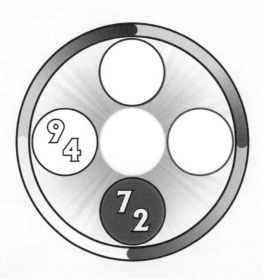

*When a man does a piece of work which is admired by all
we say that it is wonderful;
but when we see the changes of day and night, the sun, the moon,
and the stars in the sky, and the changing seasons upon the earth,
with their ripening fruits,
anyone must realize that it is the work
of someone more powerful than man.*

—Chased-by-Bears

This Signature contains dates of birth with the Numbers

7 and/or **2**
9 and/or **4**

The birthdates July 2, 1994; October 4, 1972; February 9, 1974; April 2, 1929; and July 27, 1949, are all examples of the South–West Signature, but there are many additional combinations that are possible.

At the heart of this Signature lies a brilliant combination: vibrancy with ambition. With this combination, you have the ability to not only set a good example but to also contribute to changes in the world. However, it is necessary that you make a conscious decision to do so; all imaginable life goals are within reach. And you will reach goals that mere mortals are unlikely to achieve.

This Signature offers a broad palette of opportunities on your road to self-actualization. From passionate researcher to successful painter, brilliant techno-geek to clever attorney, you will always reach your goal as long as you use your head and are assertive. Depending on the intensity of the Units of the West (**9**/**4**), those around you may see your quest as ranging anywhere from prim and proper to downright ruthless. Partners and colleagues who are more teamwork-oriented might also suffer due to the bossiness that can come with this Signature. Since you are often unaware of your effect on the outside world, try to consider how such behavior can be harmful.

The South pursues its intentions successfully with an inborn vibrancy. This Signature finds it difficult when a goal is not reached, and if the Center of Gravity is located in the South, self-criticism and objective analysis of events are also difficult. Perhaps you automatically blame and fight others. But this battle is merely an outer symptom of an inner battle between the hermit who wants to do everything alone (and realizes that this is impossible) and the power broker who realizes that others are needed in order to be successful.

People with this Signature develop great skills when handling other people's money and their own, since a healthy financial cushion at work and at home is very important to people of the South–West. Still, there are times when they find themselves short on funds—though not because they are really lacking in assets. It's just a subjective feeling of having too little. In addition, they often do not realize that they are spending beyond their means. Every Signature contains its own life challenges, and this is one for South–West.

On its own, this spendthrift tendency would not be all that bad, but there is a second challenge that could turn it into a serious problem. This is the South–West aversion to learning anything new. The North (❻/❶), which is missing in this Signature, is responsible for keeping curiosity alive despite the trap of belief, dogma, and conviction. If you don't already, you need to compensate for this lack immediately. To do this, you could take some interesting adult-education courses or incorporate the black and blue colors of the North into your clothing, home, and workplace. The choice of color can help you immensely. However, it would be best in your case to learn the art of listening, which connects you to the world, and opens new vistas and doors of opportunity.

The children of this Signature stand out for their vibrancy and mathematical ability. Their tendency to show a violent temper should not be punished. Instead, meet it with a lot of love and understanding. (Punitive actions do not work in this case—and never do, in our opinion.) The scared child will remember these chastening corrections and, depending on later development, he or she might even harbor thoughts of revenge. It would be better to set a good example for the South–West child, which is far more effective than punishment.

With this Signature, it is vital to keep negative energies from gaining the upper hand. The materialistic times we live in do not make things easier, but winning by hook and by crook is not really satisfying. It is best to lovingly make use of the talents provided by this Signature instead of exploiting the weaknesses of others.

The sooner the missing Stations—North, East, and Center—are complemented, the better and healthier the development of this Signature moving forward. This balance can be obtained in many ways: using color wisely, meditating, listening closely, and so on. It would be advantageous to be diligent about including the color green in your food. Green invites the intuition of the East into your soul, and you can never eat too many vegetables or salads! The weak points of this Signature are the liver, head, and heart, and an appropriate lifestyle would consist of regular detoxification and healthy exercise. Detox teas, springtime diets, and other cleansing practices would be of great advantage.

If you have any children with this Signature, you will have plenty of time to do the above. Children with a ❾ in this Signature need little training; the deciding factor is having a good role model. South–West children love the feeling of having achieved everything on their own (including the wholeness of their being), even as adults.

North–West

Strong will and a clear vision– great achievements are within reach

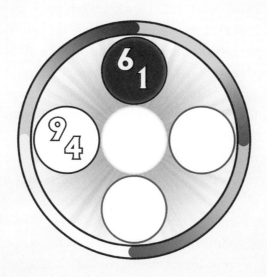

Dare what no one dares.
Say what no one is saying.
Dare to think what no one is thinking.
Finish what no one has started.
Stand back when everybody cheers.
Don't jeer when they all scoff.
Dare to give when everybody holds back.
Bring light when all is dark!

—Lothar Zenetti
(translated by Thomas Poppe)

This Signature contains dates of birth with the Numbers

⑥ and/or **①**
⑨ and/or **④**

The birthdates September 4, 1961; April 9, 1991; June 16, 1964; January 1, 1949; and September 19, 1916, are all examples of the North–West Signature.

When a date of birth combines both the North and the West, this creates a strong combination of assertiveness, discipline, and willpower. The **⑥** and **①** provide boundless energy, and the same holds true for the **⑨** and the **④**. Together, they form a power that can overcome every conceivable obstacle. People with this Signature are receptive, deep, determined, creative, and success-oriented. In principle, all doors are open to them, the Signature is suitable for a broad range of professions, from inventor to politician, journalist to craftsman, writer to scientist.

There is, however, one minor flaw. The empty East (**❽/❸**) prevents bearers of this Signature from developing empathy toward their friends, partners, and travel companions unless they see learning intuition and compassion as a way to further their success—the end that justifies the means. This is not meant in a derogatory way; it is simply what makes the North–West Signature tick. And when the Center of Gravity is in the West, this is always the case. To the outside, this behavior can appear inconsiderate and egotistical, especially if the powers of the North (**⑥** or **①**) do not have a chance to live out their special characteristics, richness of ideas, and vision. The result is sometimes a rigid, unbearable character—a sad development, especially in light of the plethora of talents that come with this Signature. While the bearer's intentions are rarely unfriendly, meditating daily and learning to listen improves the situation tremendously—and these practices are some of the keys to happiness for the people of the North–West.

Children with this Signature are frequently doing battle with everyone around them, but this will improve with maturity into adulthood. Since these children know what they want at an early age, they are not easy to raise. The trick is to simply let them be. This does not mean ignoring or neglecting them. Rather, you should accept early on that they are independent, and let them go their own way.

Parents who have many children, and nurses and caretakers who work in pediatric units, can attest to the fact that even babies can be strong-willed. Children can make far-reaching decisions much sooner than we may be aware of, although some parents (and even psychologists!) might assume that the little ones do not know yet what they are doing. Looking closer with an open mind will tell a different story, however. For these children, it is best if you set age-appropriate boundaries and chores with a flexible schedule. Otherwise, remain generous. Our children are not our property; they belong to themselves and to another Power. And having a smothering parent is especially unbearable to a child of this Signature.

In adulthood, this Signature will not tolerate being patronized; its bearers are straightforward and firm (and those in their surroundings will feel it all the more!). Incorrigibility may become a lifelong theme. When this is the case, learning takes place as a result of painful experience instead of prudent insight and foresight.

When children of this Signature have problems in school, it is rarely because they are unable to learn. Mostly, these highly intelligent children are simply bored. They also show excellent physical prowess. Many of their peers are envious of such a concentration of talents, which automatically predisposes North–West children to being outsiders. Compassionate adults and caregivers sometimes feel obligated to make up for the apparent "injustice" with extra attention, spoiling these children as consolation. Then they are surprised when their efforts cause more aggression. What this Signature really needs is recognition and respect rather than pity. And once you as the parent of such a child have figured out the dynamics, family life should be more relaxed all around.

Black and white are the colors of this Signature, whose world is also black and white: "If you don't love me, you hate me." Not every person can deal with this mind-set in a relaxed fashion. Hence, separations are not uncommon. The missing Center (0/5) becomes painfully obvious when compromises are difficult to achieve. The empathy of the East (8/3) is also absent, and the cheerful vibrancy and light-heartedness of the South (❼/❷) are nowhere to be seen. When this Signature expresses slight displeasure, it can come across as rage, so solid, stable business connections are established far more often than warm friendships.

The colors of the missing Stations—yellow, green, and red—help balance this Signature. The bottomless creativity (inventiveness) of the North will blossom once the special characteristics of the East, South, and Center are at least partially incorporated into this Signature's tool chest. We recommend using yellow around the house—on the walls or in the curtains, tablecloth, or bed linens. For green, the focus could be food or indoor plants. For public occasions, red should be used (maybe in form of a thin red string on the wrist). Having a missing South sometimes results in feeling inferior, even when everything is fine on the surface and success is at hand. So, wear a lot of red as medicine to cure the "imagined" defect.

Those who have this Signature should use its gifts and aim high, passing their significant abilities to the East and the South. Do this without ego and disconnect, and with the feeling that all is right with the world as long as one hand washes the other.

North–Center

Vision and the patient power of the Center–
a large trove of knowledge to hand out

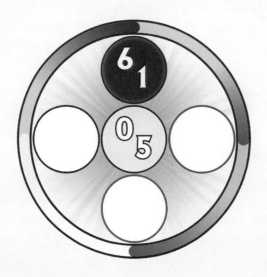

Work like you don't need the money,
Love like you've never been hurt,
Dance like nobody's watching,
Sing like nobody's listening,
Live like it's heaven on earth.
                                    —Mark Twain

This Signature contains dates of birth with the Numbers

❻ and/or ❶
⓪ and/or ⑤

The birthdates June 1, 1950; January 5, 1961; May 16, 1955; October 5, 1966; and January 10, 2005, are all examples of the North–Center Signature, but there are many additional Number combinations that also lead to this Signature.

If one's birthdate contains the ❻ or ❶ combined with the ⓪ or ⑤, the bearer will receive vital foresight when he or she awakens this special talent. The Numbers of the North stand for clear relationships, ambition, intellect and intelligence, determination, and the thirst for knowledge. The Numbers of the Center provide creative thinking, a willingness to make sacrifices, sympathy, reason, and patience. This Signature's combination is ideal for implementing various projects and ideas, especially regarding any form of publicity. The Center of the Birthday Wheel provides the North with grounded stability—the starting block, gas station, and rest area for trips into the unknown. This combination also portends luck. Only dreary childhood events that parch the soul could turn this Signature into a failure.

Sometimes, the empty West makes itself known when big ideas turn out to be castles in the sky. This does not necessarily have anything to do with the genuine quality of the idea. Instead, it is the often long road from concept to realization that reveals a hidden impatience in the Signature, despite the balancing quality of the Center. The fact that an idea cannot be realized almost immediately after its birth is hard to accept for the North–Center. If this is your personal Signature, you might want to look early on in the creative process for a business partner or colleague whose Signature has the Numbers of the West (❾/❹) and to whom you can pass on your knowledge for project completion. It is advisable, however, to keep an eye on the West and have safeguards in place. The West sometimes has a way of becoming independent; then your idea is no longer your own. But there is no need to be mistrusting. It is enough to formalize contracts and use security measures from the beginning.

This Signature does not lack empathy because the Center always balances by effectively filling the void in the East; you are more likely to feel the missing South (❼/❷). This can result in the feeling that you are not being taken seriously—that you are being overlooked or passed over—even when none of this is actually so. Some people with this Signature may receive applause but at the same moment think, "They don't really mean it. I don't deserve this." Although this is frequently a subjective feeling, if you are a bearer of the North–Center, it would not hurt to be assertive about your North–Center presence so that you might see progress in your life.

An unusually large number of children with this Signature are bookworms. They become so engrossed in reading that the world around them fades away, no matter what is going on. The child with this Signature needs good friends with the North in their birthdates, or the friendships are unlikely to last. The North–Center child's seeming withdrawal from the world is often seen as rejection and indifference. It becomes even more problematic when the bookworm is labeled "stuck up" because reading has inevitably given him or her more knowledge. He or she can be quickly labeled as boring, too.

You can see how misinformation incites people's prejudice. The key is for all involved to gain some insight and understanding about the other. Many politicians could benefit from paying attention to other views. If they did, the world would have far fewer problems. However, servants of the state frequently have their own agenda which might not surface until they have been voted out of office. Yet, it could be so simple. "By their fruits, you shall know them."

What can you do to balance the missing Stations? Pay attention to conquering the West so that your brilliant ideas don't remain daydreams and wishful thinking. To understand the West, it is sufficient to take evening classes about your special interests; wear a lot of white to meetings initially. A touch of red is also useful. For men, a thin bracelet made from red wool or leather works well. Wisely chosen colors are highly effective for balancing and complementing energies and characteristics that are missing.

Black is the color you should avoid, however, especially if your Signature's Center of Gravity is located in the North. Yellow, the color of the Center, is rarely useless or burdensome, unless you have only one Number in the North and all others are in the Center (for example, May 6, 1950). In that case, yellow should be used sparingly in day-to-day life. By using such simple tricks and having a healthy portion of self-love, you can build something beautiful with this Signature, to the benefit of you and all.

East–Center

The empathy and the harmony of the Center–
moving along a good path

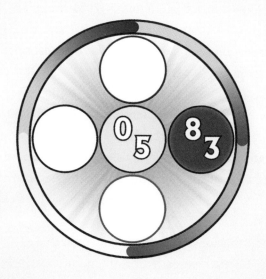

When the bee collects honey
it does not spoil the beauty or scent of the flower.
So let the sage settle in himself and wander as he wills.

—Gautama Buddha

This Signature contains dates of birth with the Numbers

8 and/or **3**
0 and/or **5**

The birthdates March 8, 1950; August 3, 1985; March 5, 1958; March 8, 1908; and March 3, 1980, are all examples of the East–Center Signature. There are only a few more possible Number combinations that lead to this Signature, making it a fairly rare combination on the Birthday Wheel.

Can there be too much of a good thing in life? The thought crosses your mind when you look at the energies that this Signature imparts to its bearers. Helping professionals such as healers, physicians, musicians, farmers, and gardeners (people often considered to have dream professions) are all at home in this Signature, as their characteristics are already present: musicality, empathy, patience, creativity, selflessness, perseverance, caring, and reason.

At first glance, this looks like a well-equipped starter kit for an interesting life journey. However, empathy for others can be overly developed—so much so that your own needs and healthy egotism get shortchanged. The feeling that you cannot go your own way leads to the decision not to follow your own happiness. This underestimation of the self happens quite frequently as a result of overbearing parents, who stifle dream jobs and other opportunities by badmouthing and forbidding them. As a result, the bearer of this Signature may also be effected physiologically and even fall ill.

Talents, yearnings, and wishes are not given to us arbitrarily. On the contrary, they are *destined* to be expressed in our lives. If this Signature decided to be born into the calculating coolness of a success-oriented family, he or she might end up being an outsider at home, and it is very painful to be misunderstood there. Although living in harmony is not equally important to everyone, in this instance, it is often perceived as vital.

The wonderful thing about the Code is that it is never too late for change, growth, and true progress; living is a constantly evolving work of art. Knowing this makes life easier instantly, enabling us to rethink our life's path. And we do not have problems because certain situations exert pressure on us; problems do not create problems. These situations occur because we keep reacting to them the same way over and over again. It is our reaction, our thinking, and our emotions that have to change. Ask yourself, "Do I have a problem because the glass is already half empty, or should I be happy and content because the glass is still half full?" Situations change when our reactions to them change.

If you have problems saying and pursuing what is dear to your heart, simply choose a different approach. Do you have to be sure of your good intentions to take an action if you do not get outside permission first? If the answer is no, then the time has come to take this step into life. Your loved ones, colleagues, and others might initially feel offended because they are not accustomed to this type of behavior from you. But is this not the same way others have always dealt with you—by presenting you with complete facts, albeit ones that were not always what your heart wanted? Taking a new path—the one that is meant for you—is your responsibility *now*. And this path is actually easy to find: it is the one that fills you with happiness.

Because you may avoid what you subjectively perceive as crude and impolite in many situations (saying a straightforward "No," for example), you may be inadvertently inviting others to make demands of you. Learn to fight back without offending. It would be a crime toward yourself and all of nature if you did not acquire this ability. Not only is it a big waste when good talents and abilities are allowed to wither away, but it is also a sure way to bring on illness and misfortune.

From now on, your blockages should be a thing of the past. If you feel that you are being overlooked too often, start using more red in your clothing, even if you are male. Promise yourself that you will shine in white from now on at business meetings. You should also deliberately include black and blue in your day-to-day life. Red, white, and black are the ideal balance for your missing Stations, and you can immerse yourself in these colors at the office, at home, or even in your car. Green and yellow are not as welcome, but you can use the colors of your Signature sparingly if you like. Remember that these colors also have an effect when you ingest them—a fact that you can now use productively.

Perhaps you can better understand now that birthdates or events like May 8, 1988, August 5, 1988, or May 8, 1955, are easy to remember but require substantial balancing of their overly strong energies. Even a sensitive person will become aggressive when too much is expected of the "good child."

If you are a person of the East–Center, actively use your insight and wisely chosen colors to eliminate many insecurities. Stage fright before a speech, butterflies at parent-teacher night at school, social jitters at a local town hall meeting—all can be a thing of the past.

There are many people who have a lot less to say than you do, and it would be a shame if your words fell victim to the limitations of your Signature. Your time has come. Allow everyone to share in your nobleness of heart. Take some time to reread the sections about the Numbers of the Center and the East in part 2. Then read about your missing Stations and watch as the circle of the Birthday Wheel closes, throwing your world aright.

South–Center

A cheerful disposition connects with the desire for harmony–
a happy road

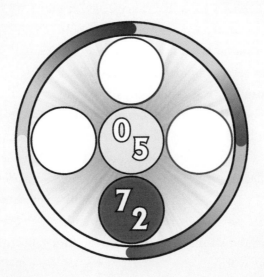

You know in virtue of what you are;
and what you are depends on three factors:
what you've inherited,
what your surroundings have done to you,
and what you've chosen to do with your inheritance.
—Aldous Huxley, *Time Must Have a Stop*

This Signature contains dates of birth with the Numbers

7 and/or **2**
0 and/or **5**

The birthdates May 27, 1950; February 2, 1972; July 5, 1952; May 7, 1902; and February 5, 2000, are all examples of the South–Center Signature. There are several other Number combinations that can create this Signature, but they are relatively few in comparison to other Signatures.

The Signature South–Center offers a special challenge to its bearers, depending on where the Center of Gravity is located. Does the South dominate? Is there a balance, or is there a strong Center (does the year or the decade contain a **0**, for example)? If the Center of Gravity is in the South (**7**/**2**), we are dealing with a spitfire, and it would be useless to slow or tie them down. They tackle everything in life with a vengeance. People with this Signature are noticed in public. They tend to achieve special things, pulling off tricks and stunts that would be too time consuming or intricate for the rest of the world.

For this Signature to be happy in life, and for us to enjoy their many great deeds in harmonious succession, it is especially important that their inner life philosophy is in line with their chosen profession. Fortunately, it is no longer that difficult to change careers and acquire a new set of skills that allow us to go a different way when we have reached a dead end. In the past, it was not nearly that simple, as the number of choices was limited, especially in rural areas. Today, the artistic side of this Signature can assert itself more easily and find its niche much sooner. The time is ripe for mavericks like you to find their place, so look for your unique spot if you want to thrive.

In order to fruitfully activate all abilities with long-term success, the South–Center Signature needs colleagues, attorneys, advisers, or a confidante with a **9** or **4**. This is due to the fact that the Signature is a relative stranger to sound business decisions—someone who does not plan and calculate down to the penny before taking a risk. On the other hand, there is a good reason for the old German adage "gelernt ist gelernt" ("You know what you know"). If you are not as coolheaded as the West, you can still teach yourself some survival skills. The advantage here is that you do not need a "manager." Instead, you just need to look for suitable partners who can compensate for your lack of analytical business sense so that you don't have to waste your time on such things.

The Center powers of your Signature ensure that you do not particularly feel a hole where you are missing a Station, and the understanding that comes with your Center makes conquering those empty Stations easier. In many cases, this is enough compensation to create harmony in the Birthday Wheel. If not, it is advisable that you reread the information about your South and Center Numbers on pages 53 and 73. After that, take the time to devote yourself to the missing Stations—West (❾/❹), North (❻/❶), and East (❽/❸). This will bring clarity into your life, and your subsequent steps will be much, much easier.

After reading the text, you will probably find that you do not miss each absent Station with the same intensity. Wherever you experience a special void, where the characteristics described are totally alien to you, first integrate more of the Station's associated color into your life. This is a simple and highly effective method. For example, do you have a problem putting yourself in the shoes of your children so that you better understand their actions? You are certainly not alone in this, but if you bring more green into your life, the situation can change. And listen more while learning to withhold your opinion. This is another important key to your child's heart (and to the hearts of all others).

Life is not easy for children with this Signature. If their high spirits are constantly being suppressed, they will give in to the pressure sooner or later and potentially miss their life's purpose as a consequence. Be careful when reining in that temperament! It would be much better to steer your child's strong powers in the right direction. Children with a South–Center Signature need a lot of outlets.

You often find top athletes and adventure seekers with this Signature; their endurance is endless. Nothing takes too long for them, and nothing is too steep, too deep, or too heavy. They were born with a love of testing their limits, agility, and body control. Professional dancers, acrobats, circus performers, magicians, and deep-sea divers are just a few of the extreme professions that they can excel at more easily than other people.

Unfortunately, there are hardly any of these funny, cheerful children around—at least not yet. Their last year in the twentieth century was 1977. But there's no need to worry. The year 2000 brought them back to us again, and some are already in school and on their way to young adulthood. If you need proof of the wonderful work of the Code, have a look at these students; you will notice the difference.

The children of the South–Center will bring us great pleasure with their Numbers. Many stubborn, greedy, arrogant, and selfish politicians, scientists, physicians, and school principals of the ❶❾th century will soon be obsolete, and more intelligent up-and-comers will have the vision to make a clean sweep of this male-dominated world that is often driven by hot air and false pride. Of course, not all will be bearers of this special Signature, so our top priority should be to raise *all* of today's children with plenty of love. Then, with the help of the South–Center children, they will have a chance to rise above the indifference and prejudice of the past to work toward true cooperation between neighbors and nations.

West–Center

Headed toward success under your own power and with patience–
boundaries to the unknown might be crossed

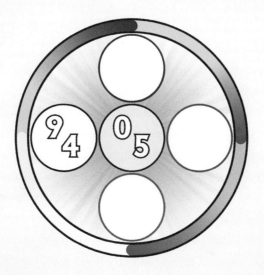

If your daily life seems poor, do not blame it;
Blame yourself that you are not poet enough to call forth its riches;
For the Creator, there is no poverty.

—Rainer Maria Rilke

This Signature contains dates of birth with the Numbers

9 and/or **4**
0 and/or 5

The birthdates April 5, 1940; September 4, 1950; April 9, 1945; May 5, 1994; and September 4, 2005, are all examples of the West–Center Signature, which is relatively rare.

The West–Center Signature promises a heavily results-oriented life where success in the visible, material sense is in the foreground. For these people, having it all is very important. This might sound selfish at first, but it isn't necessarily. This Signature does not produce whiners and crybabies; its bearers create what they need without much fuss. They go their way, self-confident and self-sufficient, and know how to help themselves without annoying those around them. They are men and women of action.

Are there many emotions invested in this Signature's situation? As a partner of a West–Center person, you must understand that he or she might occasionally regard feelings as frivolous sentimentality. In the presence of such emotions, West–Center individuals may feel that what really matters in life is not being taken seriously.

Bearers of this Signature need longer periods of retreat, and this should not be seen as indifference or rejection. Rather, it should be recognized as vital for their mental health. Often, these people use this time to figure out something new—maybe an advancement for family or society. Inventors and extreme athletes have the West–Center Signature. When these people are in control of machines, motorcycles, cars, and the like, they seem to become one with the dangerous machinery; the machine becomes an extension of their bodies.

This Signature does not require a lot of public recognition. For this reason, an inventor rarely makes a public appearance, feeling downright uncomfortable in social situations. You say you have this Signature but enjoy the public? In this case, you started conquering the empty North and South of your Signature early on in life. It might have happened in school if you had a teacher who emphasized making speeches and presentations in front of the entire class, but you were surely not born this way.

In this Signature, the Center ensures that you are happy with yourself, and you frequently arrange your life alone. You know your priorities and preferences, obtaining what is necessary but rarely at the expense of others. Although there may be an occasion when someone might suffer under your loner mentality, it will not be so extreme that you and your counterpart will become very conscious of it.

It is an extremely worthwhile task for the West–Center Signature to compensate for the empty North (❻/❶) and East (❽/❸). You may believe you can do without the latter especially—and often with passion—because speaking about your feelings and getting to know the entire breadth of human emotions is not among your strengths. If this is the case, you should interrupt this reading and go to page 41 to reread the chapter about the East. You can still reject the information after reading it, but a second review can't hurt.

The South (❼/❷) is also missing, and many Signatures without a South suffer from not being seen. However, this is not necessarily the case for a West–Center Signature. The strong West tends to get what it needs, and then has no further wishes; this Signature is no stranger to self-sufficiency. But if you feel or realize that attention is nice to have, use the color red as a good first step. Its bold inner energy represents the South and awakens the powers at home there. It also sends a cosmic invitation to vibrancy and enthusiasm. Alternatives to wearing red are numerous, from a small red rug to towels, vases, flowers, glasses, sheets, or pictures. Or you could wear a subtle red string or leather band around your wrist. A red car has a different effect on your soul plan than a white one. There are many possibilities if you make red your favorite color.

Green can also provide many benefits. The Signature of the East gets far in life by showing understanding for others and empathy for people in difficult situations. Consider carrying a green stone with you at all times in order to harness the empathetic qualities of this Cardinal Point. Minerals and precious stones of all colors are popular not only for their rarity but also because they compensate for energies we are lacking. Subconsciously, we know this and purchase what we need. (We should all listen more to our inner voice.)

When someone radiates an easygoing outer contentment, as many with this Signature do, it does not mean that deep down he or she is totally content. "No one knows what's inside," is a phrase that will ring true for many people with this Signature. Sometimes we search in vain for the key to a profound change for the better and remain stuck in an unsatisfactory situation. You say you recognized yourself in what we just said? Then starting tomorrow, you should begin working with colors. You will soon see that everything will move much better. Doors will open to rooms that your Signature had not known until now, and the adventure will be well worth it.

North–South

Joy in discovery and passing on the good news–
living the adventure

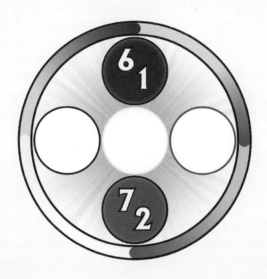

The miracle of creation is so abundant
That its beauty will never end.
Creation is here,
It is within you,
And it always has been.
The world is a miracle.
The world is magic.
The world is love.
And it is here, now.
    —Iroquois prayer of gratitude

This Signature contains dates of birth with the Numbers

6 and/or **1**
7 and/or **2**

The birthdates June 16, 1972; January 17, 1961; February 27, 1927; July 1, 1971; and January 6, 1967, are all examples of the unusually dynamic North–South Signature.

This special North–South combination and its inherent energy can be found in many professions and in pioneers of many areas of life—writers, politicians, judges, architects, and philosophers. Its formula generates the momentum necessary to accomplish great things.

We certainly hope that you have a teacher with a North-South Signature at least once in your life. If you are, in fact, a teacher with these Stations in your birthdate, the odds are in your favor of being everyone's favorite. Why? You are well equipped for enlightening and illuminating those who are adventurous, enthusiastic, and inquisitive and want to learn from you. You are intelligent, courageous, sensitive, gentle, and determined.

People of this Signature have passion for their professions, healthy curiosity, and a spirit that takes joy in changes. They exude joy when entering a room, and everything becomes brighter. The two extremes of the North and the South live happily under one roof here.

The bearers of this Signature go through life ready and able to receive. Hardly anything is too difficult for them, and they somehow manage to have an appreciation for everything. They are not born businesspeople, but having the North (**6**/**1**) compensates for much. What is so likable about them is their willingness to pass on their knowledge with no strings attached. People too often choose a profession in order to hold on to a thimble full of power. Not this Signature. The bearers of the North–South find and convey their pleasure when the transfer of knowledge works, and their students understand the material. Surely you can remember one of these teachers, even though they may have been spread thin. (The other

teachers, however, taught us a valuable lesson as well; they made us determined to not become like them!)

Bearers of this Signature are unlikely to reach a top position because
they are missing the assertiveness of the West (**9**/**4**). As children, we did
not understand that there was a connection between these two things; we
hoped for a fair world. However, as adults, we have a more realistic view of
the professional world. Now we hope that people with this Signature go
on to become school principals or perhaps work in the Department of
Education. Our future would look much different if North–South people
were in management positions in education. Then we would see truly
helpful subjects that put kids on the right track being taught at school.

This Signature also produces the charismatic top athletes who become
enshrined in our collective consciousness. It is at home wherever healthy
ambition is required, especially in extreme professions like investigative
and combat journalism or healthcare organizations like the Red Cross or
Doctors without Borders. People in these fields have the courage to live the
lives that are usually only seen in movies.

Of course, you bearers of the North–South Signature have your limits.
Your Cardinal Points bring a lot of vitality to your personality, but you
sometimes build spectacular castles in the clouds—unless the moderating
and grounded influence of attorneys, managers, or secretaries can bring you
back to earth. If you decide to go into business for yourself, you will be well
received by everyone. However, you may not feel so welcome in the world
anymore when there is no money in the bank at the end of the month.

Such people sometimes need to go out into the world in order to
return to find their true calling. The bottom line is that they sometimes
lack understanding outside of their immediate interests. For example, it
often does not matter to them that these days music is being blasted all
over the place (a destructive force that has yet to be recognized). But this
one-sidedness can be a good thing, because it means that this Signature
does not follow every trend.

If you sometimes feel the effect of the missing West (**9**/**4**), East (**8**/**3**),
and the Center (**0**/**5**) in your day-to-day life, you can compensate and

harmonize your traits by using the colors white, green, and yellow. Make sure to incorporate these colors into your wardrobe, food, workplace, and home. You can learn to further understand the West by taking ongoing education classes, and you should initially wear a lot of white when attending meetings. Some green and yellow in your color palette would also be advantageous. For men, a thin green, yellow, or white wristband of wool or leather would be sufficient. Wisely chosen colors are extremely effective for balancing and complementing the empty Stations in an unobtrusive fashion, making it even easier to experience their benefits.

People of the North–South Signature tend to be likeable, interesting, and vibrant, and can be even more so—to the advantage of all—when their Stations are in balance.

East–West

Creative capability and empathetic harmony– a successful model in action

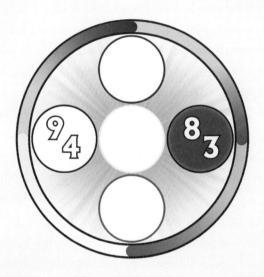

White people are too restless!
They relentlessly rush back and forth and worry about
How they could worry and rush even more.
They hurry through life, so that they have no time
To admire its beauty or to feel deep thoughts.
I am happier than the white people
Because I do not fret about these things
And if I worry about my belongings
I give them away.

—Hosteen Klah, Navajo medicine man

This Signature contains dates of birth with the Numbers

8 and/or **3**
9 and/or **4**

The birthdates September 3, 1983; August 4, 1949; April 8, 1993; March 9, 1934; and September 3, 1984, are all examples of the East–West Signature. This is a rare Signature that will occur next on March 3, 2034.

Two worlds truly collide here, when capability, ambition, creativity, and astuteness meet moderation, closeness to nature, and harmony. Each Cardinal Point on its own is an extreme, but together, they play a song that could climb high on the charts. Bearers of this Signature are needed everywhere and can be deployed almost anywhere; their success is virtually pre-programmed. Of course, a few things need to be done and have to happen first. The gentle East (**8**/**3**) needs to ensure that success does not go to one's head, making for too much high-spiritedness.

Depending on where the Center of Gravity is, the bearer of this Signature might exhibit musical talent or healing abilities, but without any romantic undertones. Instead, these traits are combined with the West's (**9**/**4**) ability to promote oneself.

Children with this Signature know early on in life what they want. They do not need an overly protective mother or a domineering father to constantly rein in their enthusiasm and independence. In daily life, these children manage well. However, without boundaries of any kind, they can become quite a handful, getting on people's nerves. They may be convinced that their pushiness is nothing more than giving the attention that is desired, but they will learn the difference over time.

In adulthood, East–West people sometimes shortchange their private lives, as they have little understanding for a life that revolves around lots of parties and reveling. The same goes for appearance. Style and fashions have not mattered since they were young, and they make it simple for themselves. Buying timeless, quality clothing is good enough.

If the Center of Gravity of this Signature is located in the West, it is necessary to keep a watchful eye on the tendency to exploit people financially. Be careful that you do not take unfair advantage of anyone around you. This Signature has the capability to do this, which is often apparent in day-to-day life. On the other hand, if the East outweighs the West, you run the risk that your overly cautious nature will not appreciate the abilities of the West and will suppress them. If you see these traits in yourself, you can intervene to rectify them in a timely fashion now. A first step would be to avoid the color white if your West is too strong. If the East dominates, stay clear of the color green.

The missing Center (5 / 0) often creates an inner unrest that cannot be explained. It is difficult to pinpoint its origin, much like the feelings we experienced during puberty. The color yellow could do a lot of good in this case and would also provide balance. The empty North (6 / ❶), with its (latent) enthusiasm for taking steps into a new world, can be brought to life by the colors blue and black. A missing North generally interferes with the eagerness to learn new skills or broaden one's intellectual horizon if the immediate benefit is not obvious. A well-developed West can make up for this, however. If we sometimes exclude certain subjects or, more explicitly, we do not even think about them, then they will be missing in certain key situations because we do not have them in our life's tool kit.

When the South (❼ / ❷) is missing, we sometimes feel that life is passing us by, or that we are being overlooked and underappreciated. Such feelings foster unhealthy competitiveness that is destructive over time. Red clothing, food, or jewelry can ease this tendency.

The bearers of the East–West Signature are rarely drawn to public relations work; they prefer working behind the scenes. They work hard and appreciate praise and recognition, too, but not necessarily in public. This Signature is most content with a successful business life that is humane, harmonious, and financially rewarding.

One of this Signature's defining traits is its emphasis on the home, which is almost indispensable for its bearers, who literally need a nest to be completely happy. A well-furnished apartment also works as long as one truly feels secure and at home in it.

All in all, this Signature is well equipped for forging a great path in life. When you live the East–West's good traits and conquer what is missing, almost all doors in life will be open to you.

10. The Ten Triples

North–East–South

Determination, vibrancy, and compassion—
a successful triad

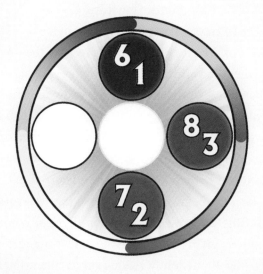

We sometimes complain about bad times,
But times are only bad
When people are bad.
Good times do not fall from heaven;
We have to create them,
Not with money and technology, but with kindness and heart.
Only good people make good times,
When goodwill reigns and when violence is silent,
When wealth is shared and when people like each other,
When there is room for a flower,
And time for a friendly word.

—Phil Bosmans
(***translated by Thomas Poppe***)

This Signature contains dates of birth with the Numbers

6 and/or **1**
8 and/or **3**
7 and/or **2**

The birthdates July 2, 1963; March 13, 1972; August 16, 1973; July 17, 1961; and June 7, 1937, are all examples of the numerous combinations possible for the North–East–South Signature.

Whether in the form of a friendly piece of advice or a stern reprimand, every child in the world sooner or later gets to hear the phrase, "Do something with your life!" If you have this Signature, consider yourself lucky because, with the abilities of these Stations, you can achieve goals effortlessly. It is rare to find such distinct and colorful characters as can be found among people with this Number combination. Whether singer, politician, physician, or freedom fighter, the women and men with these Numbers are superbly equipped to go their own way—undeterred and determined to succeed. From the very beginning, they have had the tools for the most interesting life scripts. We need to mention here, of course, that, just as with other Signatures, giving and receiving active support and encouragement are much better than simply relying on dormant talents. Good tools come to a productive life only in willing and skilled hands.

The treasure chest of this Signature's triad has it all. The East (**8**/**3**) provides patience, compassion, and perseverance to achieve seemingly unattainable goals and to realize bold dreams. The vibrancy and charisma of the South (**7**/**2**) convince other people that your way is doable and worthwhile. And the two are joined by the power of the North (**6**/**1**), with its profound capacity and determination. Fate would have to deal you a terrible hand for you to not conjure up something special from these gifts.

For one, music is in your blood. Whether you sing or play an instrument, you will have an audience. You are also a talented dancer. You should allow those around you to dance with you, so to speak, in one form or another. When it comes to the career choices open to this Signature, with the right amount of time and effort, you can learn anything (just as you can learn to sing and dance). You were born with knowledge. It is almost as if you don't have to practice in order to be perfect. Of course, another law of nature applies here: it is possible that this talent is still slumbering. You need to take the risk and bring your innate ability to the surface. Polish this treasure and make it shine.

You might be familiar with films that show children learning how to ride a bicycle, ski, dance, or ice skate; there are distinct differences in each child's absorption levels. Some practice a little at whatever the activity is, and then they have perfect form for the rest of their lives—like the ten-year-old skiers who master the mountain runs in ways that are not taught in any ski school, the teenage tennis superstars who grace Wimbledon, or the young virtuoso violinists who play in philharmonics. Others never really get the hang of it, even when they become adults. A child with the North–East–South has this special gift of "getting it." They could take piano lessons for only two years and be able to enchant you with a sound dreamscape that would take most people years and years to master. The essential message here is that if this is your Signature, you can go full throttle. The world is your oyster.

And what is the less desirable news amidst all the good news for bearers of this Signature? Two Stations are missing, namely, the balancing Center (0 / 5) and the coolheaded West (❾/❹). This essentially means that you might overshoot your mark—by a little or a lot; you savor everything to the limit. Sometimes there is simply nothing left toward the end, and you can only shake your head in disbelief because you did not see it coming (your intuitive East notwithstanding). Being well informed is half your battle. From now on, this information will make it easier for you to avoid self-created pitfalls. One of the talents of this Signature is the ability to learn. In this instance, it is rarely blocked by false pride or laziness.

What effect does the missing West have? Basically, you are very good at what you do, but others may sometimes reap your rewards. Fill this void actively and consciously; otherwise, you will be repeatedly swindled. The generous East can give away so much that it leads to irresponsible physical and financial depletion. Wear a lot of white to important appointments, as this simple trick will help you stay alert. You should also engage a good adviser who has the Numbers of the West.

There are no other dangers lurking in the wings of the North–East–South Signature. Cope with the few hurdles you have and enjoy life. And let *us* share in your successes, too. Film and TV now make this easy, as many a movie star, musician, and sports figure with this Signature has made our evenings more pleasant over the past decades.

East–South–West

The joy of dreams coming to life–
a good balance of emotion and reason

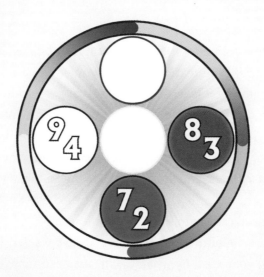

A famous sculptor was working on a marble lion.
A visitor, full of admiration, asked what the secret of his art was.
The Master answered,
"That is not that difficult,
I merely chisel away anything that does not resemble a lion."
—Traditional Arabian saying

This Signature contains dates of birth with the Numbers

8 and/or **3**
7 and/or **2**
9 and/or **4**

The birthdates September 8, 1973; July 3, 1994; April 22, 1983; August 9, 1982; and February 23, 1944, are all examples of the East–South–West Signature—a special combination with many talents.

Signatures cannot be labeled by one typical profession or one type of person. Such typecasting would never do justice to the interplay of active support and conditioning—of decisions based on free will and subconscious mental impasses. There are countless influences at play here: upbringing, role models, possibilities, and temptations. Many factors, even trivial ones, influence us long-term. Still, the Signature of the East–South–West seems to have a strong correlation to the acting profession.

If this is your Signature and you have always wanted to act on some level, then fulfill your wish by whatever means necessary. You say you are not so young anymore and are already on a different path? There is always a need for older actors! If acting does not grab your interest, however, do not worry; this is by no means the only talent you can manifest. If you reread the description of your Numbers in part 2, you will see that you also have many other qualities. For example, the influence of the South (**7**/**2**) ensures that you are popular with everyone, for you brighten the day with your contagious enthusiasm. Not only is your glass half full, but those around you learn to be less pessimistic as well. And your day really comes to life after work. When you have to turn down an invitation to a party (which you rarely do voluntarily), the party is only half as fun.

Since the East (**8**/**3**) stands for great empathy, you usually know how to express it in the right proportions; you rarely make a wrong decision. Having the innate ability to clearly discern where you are (or aren't) needed and for how long makes life much easier for you both personally and professionally. You need to be cautious, however, if you have a pronounced Center of Gravity in the East. What is well meaning could turn into too much of a good thing, giving a new meaning to the old proverb "The road to hell is paved with good intentions." Your house and your heart can be open doors to a flood of impressions and influences because you have not learned how to say no. The ability to say no may have been pushed back by formative childhood influences but must now be learned anew. You will receive help from the power of the West.

The West (❾/❹) sharpens your business sense. Just as a reminder, the ❾ imparts a greater ability to manage money than does the ❹, which promotes mechanical and manual skills. Should you actually have a profession in which you use your acting talent, it is likely that you need a stand-in only during the most dangerous scenes and stunts.

The empty Center (0 / 5) will cause you to lose your balance when you misjudge the available energies; that is part of your life theme. For example, you may think you don't pass muster, your successes notwithstanding. Let us assure you that there is no need for such self-doubt.

Although your Signature has an empty North (❻/❶), your special trio of the other Stations usually compensates successfully for this void. For example, you might feel the absence of the North when you find yourself lacking endurance during intense mental tasks; you have always had a different way of learning. This was not always easy for your teachers to accept, especially for that certain type of teacher who believed cramming rote knowledge was the only way to learn. There are many people who do not understand that someone can learn and understand almost anything without extensive studying. From now on, simply ignore such enviers. Becoming a teacher might be a good career choice for you, especially if you have discovered the true joy of sharing knowledge. If not, learn how to search for it yourself!

Your Signature is not conducive to your doing things alone, however. Solitude is not your way, and a good team can often accomplish more anyway. From the very beginning, you provide the required fairness needed for successful teamwork, even if it is buried under prior disappointments.

When you find yourself in a situation where you feel inertia, give the colors black and blue a try. Emerging in black and appearing in blue will require little change but provide a substantial long-term effect.

There is much in life that must first be awakened and used; that is what we are here for. When we really think about it, the happiest "coincidences" in life turn out to be nothing more than reaping what we have sown. Use your strong personality! Whatever you need is available to you.

North–South–West

With endurance and wisdom to visible success–achievement and beyond

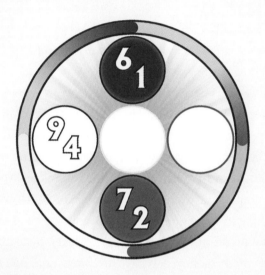

In order to live, you must savor life.

I don't mean the self-indulgence that makes so many people ill

And enslaves and plunges them into misery.

In order to savor life, you must be free

Free of greed, free of envy, free of passions

that tear you apart and destroy you

If you can savor life, you can laugh

You are happy, you are thankful that the sun rises for you every morning.

You can be delighted over a soft bed and a warm apartment

You meet friendly people

You encounter God's friendship in every smile,

In every flower, in every kind word, in each hand, in each hug.

If you can savor small things leisurely,

then you are living in a garden of bliss.

—**Phil Bosmans**
(**translated by Thomas Poppe**)

This Signature contains dates of birth with the Numbers

6 and/or **1**
7 and/or **2**
9 and/or **4**

The birthdates September 16, 1972; January 4, 1967; July 2, 1991; February 7, 1941; and June 9, 1962, are all examples of the many possible combinations of the North–South–West Signature.

"What is success?" There have been countless answers for that since the beginning of time. It is not just beauty that is in the eye of the beholder; if you look closely, success also means something different to everyone. The bearers of this Signature, however, tend to have one thing in common: it is fine for success to be in the form of something tangible. We often hear that there are more important things in life than money. However, the saying "There is no shame in having money" is absolutely true as well. This Signature does not pay attention to either saying, however. Instead, its catchphrase is "You don't talk about money. You have it." Rarely does one meet a bearer of the North–South–West Signature who has chronic money worries. They have it, use it, and love it. End of story.

The bearers of this Signature also land on their feet when they fall. As bystanders, we may not see how often they fall because these people can be very discreet, but they will make sure that we catch the successful landing. You often get the impression that dealing successfully with problems is a breeze for them. Inventive, quick-witted, and enterprising, North–South–West people move smoothly in any environment.

What if you do not feel this way when looking into a mirror or examining your past? Rest assured that you have it in you! This ability is only waiting to be revived.

At the same time, your readiness for risk is far outside the realm of most people's. Adventure is not a foreign word to you, but it is always limited to a calculated risk. You reach almost every goal with cool calculation. This is one of the hidden dangers, one of the life themes of this Signature.

Cool calculation sometimes ices over people of the North–South–West, and their success goes to their heads. Since they always land on their feet, learning from their mistakes isn't a priority, and they may show a certain "No one can stop me!" arrogance, thereby alienating people. When the West is overemphasized in comparison to the other two Cardinal Points (for example, when a ❾ and ❹ are in the date of birth), people of this Signature will exude greater negative reactions than just a shake of the head.

If you are an East–South–West person, balancing the missing Stations— Center (⓪/❺) and East (❽/❸)—might cause you problems, but it is more likely that the people around you will have problems with your perceived arrogance. It seems that sometimes you do not feel that anything is missing in your life or that anything needs to be improved. If you measure success by the growth of your bank account, you are right at home in these current times. True success has nothing to do with money, however; that much is certain. Money is a necessity, and even though it is crucial to use it wisely, the amount is unimportant. This is one of your life lessons.

Live your abilities, but also take care of the powers of the Center and the East in order to become whole. You do not make it easy for other people to express their emotions toward you. Bearers of this Signature sometimes confuse feelings with "weakness," so feelings remain hidden. Whatever the case may be, we all can learn and understand that the suppression of feelings is akin to cutting off one's oxygen. By using the colors yellow and green, you can provide more harmony for what is out of balance in your life. And by wisely selecting the appropriate colors for your clothing, home, and food, you can influence things very quickly and effectively. Rediscovering and living by previously suppressed feelings can be a special adventure that is rewarding and enjoyable from your new vantage point.

If this is your Signature, you have a great deal of persuasive power and endurance. You are also capable of letting things lie, if necessary, and will strike when the iron is hot. If we were to give this Signature an animal symbol, the lion would surely be the perfect choice here. As such, the combative spirit of your Signature should not be blocked. If a child with this Signature is smothered or oppressed, he or she is likely to react with revenge or total resignation later in life. A doting mother is a catastrophe for this type of child. Since North–South–West children do not have the Center (the **0** / **5** stand for maternal energy), they assume for too long that they are dependent upon their mothers, and can experience feelings of rage toward themselves and others.

Therefore, it is very important that we are allowed to live our lives (and our Signatures!) by using our own intuition to create an overall, harmonious balance. We can always learn from others, and there is no harm in imitating ideals and role models. But you should only admire, never envy. People of this Signature are promised a jump-start in worldly success, but everyone has to live and walk their own path in their own time. Enjoy the success-promising of your Numbers and seize the day—every day!

North–East–West

Multitalented, persevering, and empathetic–
the medley for a good path

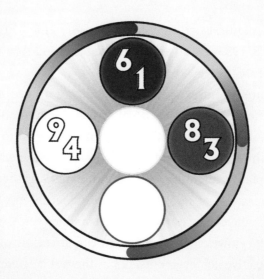

The three most difficult things for man are not acts of physical prowess or intellectual gems, but:

First: to return hatred with love

Second: to include the excluded

Third: to admit error

When these three things are mastered, life is mastered.

—Anthony de Mello

(translated by Thomas Poppe)

This Signature contains dates of birth with the Numbers

6 and/or **1**
8 and/or **3**
9 and/or **4**

The birthdates August 14, 1961; March 9, 1961; June 8, 1994; January 3, 1949; and April 6, 1983, are all examples the North–East–West Signature— the "Roof Signature" as we like to call it.

This Signature promises to bring a stabilizing influence in the lives of its bearers. Whatever they plan to do, they will achieve it. Sometimes people find it difficult to fathom why bearers of this Signature are successful at virtually anything they try, but not when you see the strengths of their fortuitous interplay of talents: a sharp mind joined together with empathy and a healthy business sense. People of this Signature mostly choose professions that provide close contact with the public (you'll find quite a few politicians here). However, they came to the attention of the public by merit of their positive achievements, not as the result of media hype or the persuasiveness of ad agencies.

With the North (**6**/**1**), this Signature is very well equipped to take on lengthy courses of study (architecture, medicine, and so on). At times these studies are not totally satisfying, leading to the pursuit of a second profession or a second calling. In this instance, the East (**8**/**3**) imparts genuine altruism, which is important for figures who have extensive contact with the public. They need to have a great deal of tact because every person they deal with is different.

It takes brains and skill, as well as vision and courage, to meet the needs of an entire nation. Campaign promises show over and over where short-lived seduction leads. Therefore, never wait for or rely on concessions and promises; if you are a North–East–West person, always use your Signature's power and self-responsibility to educate yourself. As the ancient proverb goes, "Whatever is left after a shipwreck is yours." We only truly possess our heart and mind. We are always responsible for owning it or abandoning it. Of course, multiple outside influences do affect life, but with the treasure chest provided by this Signature, you can become a wonderful, wise captain during the calm periods, gentle breezes, and storms.

The West (❹/❾) in your Signature helps you congeal your intuitions into useful action, as manual dexterity is an asset that bridges many gaps in your everyday life. An innate touch for financial affairs is also an advantage here. This Signature sometimes reveals the subtle difference between the ❹ and the ❾, whereas the ❹ enhances all motor capacities, the ❾ gives somewhat more of the ability to assert oneself and a keener sense for the world of finances.

Your missing Center (❴0❵/❺) has the potential to give you a hazy sense of dissatisfaction from existing or unrecognized problems (even if they are only imagined) that creep into your life despite your multiple successes. Again, we recommend simple but effective color remedies. Increase the presence of yellow in your daily life—in your wardrobe, on your walls, and all over your curtains. Surround yourself with yellow flowers, or use yellow bed and bathroom linens; they will create balance, and that strange feeling in the pit of your stomach will disappear. A few minutes of meditation every day—with the addition of soothing music—is also helpful.

Additionally, red would enhance your life in many ways. Since red represents the South (❼/❷), it awakens the energies at home in this Station. This does not mean that you are lacking the necessary vitality to fulfill your tasks and intentions; the missing South just makes you feel overlooked and passed by, even if that feeling is an illusion. When this happens, it is merely the empty South making itself felt. Bring the color red into your life, and the void will slowly fill. Just be careful not to overdo it. You are well equipped for the special path in your life and do not always need everything that you want at any given moment. To ask for strawberries in the winter does more damage to the world than the good that out-of-season fruit does for our bodies.

The treasure chest for your Signature has everything you need to make something special of yourself and your life—whether as a musician, politician, journalist, nursery school teacher, or business person. Furthermore, your great manual skills are equally prevalent, so who knows what fine effort you might get off the ground!

North–East–Center

Convincing, charismatic, and empathetic –
into the limelight with the energies of the Center

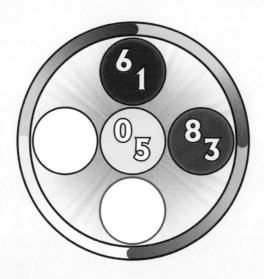

There is more than one path
That leads to life after life.
There is more than one way to love.
There is more than one path
To find the other half of our self
In another person.
There is more than one way to fight an enemy.
He who cannot love his self
Cannot love anyone.
He who cannot respect the gifts received before he was born
Cannot ever properly respect anything.

—Native American proverb

This Signature contains dates of birth with the Numbers

⑥ and/or ❶
❽ and/or ❸
⓪ and/or ⑤

The birthdates October 8, 1961; June 13, 1988; March 5, 1960; May 11, 1938; and November 13, 1950, are all examples of the North–East–Center Signature.

Attributes of the North (⑥/❶) are ambition, curiosity, vision, and fortitude. When combined with the strength of the Center (⓪/⑤), this Signature promises high levels of determination and responsibility. Add the special energies of the East (❽/❸) and empathy becomes a part of this success-promising energy, offering a solid foundation for contentment (with the exception of a few small obstacles that might become bothersome).

At times, you may have a nagging feeling that something is missing in your happiness, preventing you from settling down easily. You may have exhibited a tendency to search for this missing "something" at a relatively young age, even during childhood (if your environment and your parents were willing to cooperate). No need to worry, however; you are eminently equipped for this kind of introspection at any age.

Some caution is warranted, however. Your determined energies might cause you to overreach yourself, leading you to believe that you can overcome the obstacles in the South and the West of this Signature without any outside help. The tendency to overexert yourself arises from your mistaken belief that you must do everything on your own.

Depending on how the energies are distributed and where the emphasis is within its three Cardinal Points, this Signature can manifest self-sacrifice or even self-abandonment. If the emphasis lies in the East (if the East contains both the ❽ and ❸, for example), this can result in you wanting to learn everything in isolation. You may also be convinced that you need to know everything immediately, without allowing yourself sufficient time to learn and practice. You maintain that you should be perfect without practice, and learning the virtues of patience is imperative in this case. Children with this Signature should never be left alone without their knowledge, as this could result in mistrust, insecurity, and fear of abandonment later in life.

If the North (❻/❶) is the strongest Station of this Signature, your life orientation leans heavily toward public service, and your inherent quality of empathy (derived from the ❽ or ❸) would be extremely advantageous in many organizations or enterprises.

But be on guard. When you interact with the public and also have more than ten Units in the East, which indicates an overdeveloped sensitivity, your highly developed empathy could get out of hand and interfere with successful work. You may become too tolerant of people at work or at home who wallow in self-pity, causing stress and anger to turn inward. Often, the strength to intervene in an emotionally charged situation is lacking because it is overruled by the demands of excessive emotion; your "bad conscience" gets in the way. Remaining in a stressful environment or situation against our better judgment, however, is a formula that can result in inappropriate aggression.

The balance here is a proper mixture of the cool common sense of the North and the patience and empathy of the East. Bringing in these qualities allows you to effortlessly deal with overemphasized Cardinal Points. It might also be helpful to meditate on the following rarely considered fact: By quietly tolerating difficult people, we prevent them from learning and maturing. Some of us may never learn (or we'll learn only belatedly) that we reap what we sow, even though all of the signposts are there to lead us in the right direction.

In all the possible number combinations that make up this Signature, the Center (⓪ and ⑤) ensures balance and harmony with its special energies. And this particular Signature doesn't contain Numbers that indicate aggressive tendencies, so people of the North–East–Center should be easy to get along with. They exhibit precision, curiosity, and determination, as well as a love of music, but they need variety in their lives. They should not be stuck behind counters or desks for their entire careers.

For people of the North–East–Center, finances have a low priority. They sometimes overlook the fact that money is a necessity and may have little appreciation for those who are solely motivated by money. This might sound very noble, but those whose Signature contains a heavy emphasis on the West (❾/❹) might despair because this carefree approach is alien to them. People with this Signature rarely consider material losses as true loss; rather, they see the financial situation mainly as an opportunity to cleanse and start anew.

The missing South (❼/❷) can bring on fatigue and dreariness when bearers of the North–East–Center Signature encounter obstacles. They may experience feelings of resignation and depression, and find it difficult to free themselves from these feelings on their own. Since people with this Signature are often convinced that they can and must manage things alone, the process of freeing themselves from an emotional low is likely to be very slow. They can minimize this tendency, however, by picking the right colors for their wardrobe and surroundings. White and red are excellent choices.

Your next step should be to go over your Cardinal Points again, as these comprise your big tool box (see part 2). After that, you might carefully read about the West and the South in order to gain an understanding for what is missing. When you work to achieve balance, the circle will close—for the well-being of those around you and your own.

East–South–Center

With vibrancy and eloquence– patiently serving a good cause

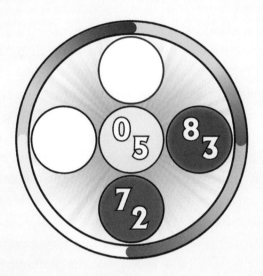

The most important hour is always now
The most important person
Is always the one standing in front of you
The most necessary greater good is love
—Meister Eckhart
(translated by Thomas Poppe)

This Signature contains dates of birth with the Numbers

⑧ and/or ③
❼ and/or ②
⓪ and/or ⑤

The birthdates March 5, 1972; August 23, 2005; February 8, 1972; July 3, 1955; and August 27, 1903, are all examples of the Signature of the East–South–Center.

The Numbers of the Center, the ⓪ and ⑤, bestow a special power on each Signature, which has a balancing, mediating, calming, and grounding effect. Whenever a Signature has a strong Center, the powers of the other Stations orient themselves more toward moderation and balance; there is no need to worry if the Center of Gravity is located in an outer Cardinal Point or if a Station is missing. In the attempt to make them your own, you need not assimilate the qualities of missing Stations as if you were born with them. The Center is always ready to help—assuming you let it.

When you were born, you were given the ability to settle conflicts. Having the ⓪ or ⑤ in your date of birth provides you with more understanding about the significance of the missing Stations. The Center is the great bridge builder.

Even a person with an extreme South—someone who was born on May ❷❷, 200❼, for example—will not lose control because the Center provides protection and balance. However, a strong South without the influence of the Center could result in periodic outbursts of rage as an ongoing element of one's character. Even with a strong Center, it is not a good idea to suppress your temperament. It is part of your path and part of your natural equipment.

With this Signature, the East (❽/❸) also provides calm and moderation. If, however, the East gains the upper hand with many Units of the ❽ or ❸, the reverse might happen. People who take care of others day in and day out are common with this Signature, but bearers might find that their own needs fall by the wayside. While this is normal for the Signature in the short term, it is not healthy in the long term. In fact, it can build up to a spectacular emotional outburst—those around will be shocked! When you get such a reaction, it's a good sign that you need to show more of your true inner self; it is not worth suppressing our true self for anyone or anything. If those around you do not accept you as you are in your daily life, it is time to wake up. "Love your neighbor as you love yourself," but remember to also love yourself as your neighbor. After a long period of self-denial, a change of mood can also happen quietly. To the outside world, this person remains understanding and sacrificing, but his or her family may detect their loved one becoming overly emotional and entirely inconsiderate. These are all signs of an overdeveloped East, and recognizing them brings you one step closer to balancing them.

Every Signature with a "live" East shows a lot of empathy and a strong capacity for compassion. Social services, nonprofit organizations, and aid projects would be doomed without the participation of at least a few people of the East. For people without an ❽ or ❸ in their dates of birth (who work in youth homes or for Child Protective Services), having well-founded theoretical knowledge might be very pragmatic, but they could find it difficult or impossible to relate to young people. Often embittered, jaded people in social professions either lack the East in their date of birth, or they have numbed it.

The East–South–Center Signature represents a vibrant, empathetic person who knows what he or she wants. The oratory skills of this Signature—the persuasive power of the South (❼/❷)—is enriching in many areas of life. After all, what good is the best product when no one is aware of its existence? Unfortunately, the oratory skills of the ❼ and ❷ can escalate into liking to hear oneself talk without giving true benefit to the listener. This is a sign of a hidden lust for power.

The missing North (❻/❶) can cause problems when beginning an undertaking since a sense of the proper sequence can be missing. The education process could also tax the patience of people who have this Signature. This does not mean they have an inability to learn; it merely means they go about things differently than others.

The missing West (**9**/**4**) can stop people with this Signature from implementing good ideas and improvements (which are often brilliant), but partners or colleagues who have the West in their birthdates could offer support in this area to the benefit of all.

To begin facing the challenge of filling in the empty Stations, colors are the fastest and easiest remedy. You should remember to use white for the missing West and blue and/or black for the missing North, and it is up to you whether you use these colors in your wardrobe, furniture, or other aspect of your home. Use your instincts, as you have plenty of them. If you have a child with this Signature and he or she always wears black, close your eyes and try to accept that this is a natural compensatory act.

Every Signature has its special qualities and its weaknesses, but the East–South–Center Signature has all the necessary abilities to conquer the missing Stations of your Birthday Wheel with ease. We wish you luck!

South—West—Center

Blazing the path for innovation—
with dedication and a feeling for timing

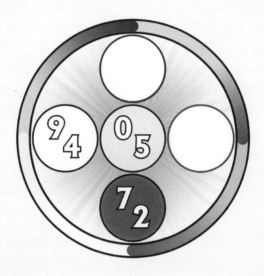

There is no divine pardon that saves you from evolution
If you want to be, you can only be in God,
He will bring you into his shelter
after you have slowly evolved through your life experiences and
have been kneaded into shape
Man takes a long time to be born.

—Antoine de Saint-Exupéry
(translated by Thomas Poppe)

This Signature contains dates of birth with the Numbers

7 and/or **2**
9 and/or **4**
0 and/or 5

The birthdates May 4, 1992; May 2, 1949; February 5, 1994; September 7, 2005; and February 5, 1974, are all examples of the South–West–Center Signature, and there are many additional Number combinations possible.

In short, the characteristics of this triad include practical thinking, a handiness with tools, and an ambitious, vibrant, and enterprising nature. As always, the presence of the Center (**0**/5) imparts a special inner strength to this Signature, and adventurous conquerors—as well as daring inventors—are at home here.

The South (**7**/**2**), the West (**9**/**4**), and the Center (**0**/5) are a fascinating combination from which real heroes emerge. Humankind as a whole would have already evolved for the better if we all had the courage to go public with our good ideas. At some point in your life, you have probably heard about or seen a new product and thought, "I thought of that years ago." The difference for people with this Signature is that they follow through on their ideas and implement them, as opposed to letting them remain just good thoughts. However, it is a long rocky road until the product is ready for the market. Many might have the idea but don't know where to begin, where to find the courage, or how to raise the money to get it market-ready. The bearers of this Signature, however, have the innate ability to see things through to completion.

The West has brought many a product into the world, and the bearers of this Signature are perfectly suited for this. However, when the Center of Gravity is located in the West, bearers may find that dollar signs wake up egotism and greed, sabotaging their success. The West always needs money and has it available most of the time. For a person of the West, it is difficult to understand that everyone does not share this same interest in money.

When hunting for new innovations of any kind, the South will provide the necessary alertness for the people of the South–East–Center, who sense needs and trends effortlessly and know what bandwagons to jump on. This talent is important—because let's be honest, what good is the best product when no one knows about it?

It isn't easy to ignore the persuasiveness of the South when a bearer of its Numbers presents and illustrates a recommendation convincingly. However, such a presentation may turn into inane chatter if the Center of Gravity is located in the South. With effort, the South–West–Center Signature can count on the assistance of the Center, which ensures that everything takes place in an orderly fashion. The presence of the Center alone makes this threesome of Cardinal Points virtually unbeatable. Without it, the South–West Signature may prove to be a safe haven for egotists.

When any Signature has a missing East (❽/❸), its bearers are likely to commit a few unpleasant blunders before learning their lesson; compassion and deep perception were not necessarily given to them at birth. The color green in clothing and around the house has a positive influence here, and spending time in nature generates the energy needed to gain insight. Then the energies of the Center help to see adventures through to successful conclusions.

The missing North can spoil the mood of the bearers of this Signature because it is hard for them to accept that there are people who might be smarter than they are. And this happens mostly when self-confidence has been shaken. The North alone does not make its bearers smarter, but people of the North are quite capable of keeping up with or actually surpassing others. While others may not notice this because they are not as competitive, bearers of the South–West–Center Signature might well be bothered by it. We all have our rough edges, and it is important to smooth them out to get life moving again. But it takes patience for coal to turn into a diamond.

If you have this Signature, and your dream of becoming a journalist has been momentarily squelched because you now know the importance of the North in such a profession, then please know that your Zodiac sign also plays a certain role here. If for you are an Air sign (Gemini, Libra, or Aquarius), for example, your mental agility will make it easier for you to cope with the special requirements of this profession and others like it.

When young people or adults with this Signature wear black, they have often chosen exactly the right color. (This information might be helpful to parents who have grown tired of seeing their kids wearing black all the time.) Green, black, and blue are the colors that propel this Signature toward happiness in life.

North–West–Center

With patience comes the success of all enterprises–
supported by the levelheaded power of the Center

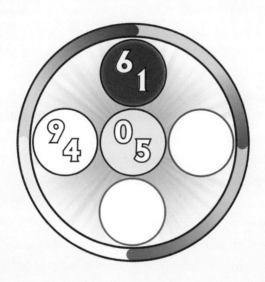

Listen to the Exhortation of the Dawn!
Look to this Day!
For it is Life, the very Life of Life.
In its brief course lie all the
Verities and Realities of your Existence.
The Bliss of Growth,
The Glory of Action,
The Splendor of Beauty;
For Yesterday is but a Dream,
And To-morrow is only a Vision;
But To-day well lived makes
Every Yesterday a Dream of Happiness,
And every Tomorrow a Vision of Hope.
Look well therefore to this Day!
Such is the Salutation of the Dawn!

—Kalidasa

This Signature contains dates of birth with the Numbers

6 and/or **1**
9 and/or **4**
0 and/or 5

The birthdates June 15, 1949; January 14, 2005; September 5, 1961; May 11, 1938; and November 13, 1950, are all examples of the North–West–Center Signature.

This Signature promises a well-developed business sense (for ventures of all kinds) with the necessary stamina and enduring patience to successfully build independent enterprises. The sharp mind of the North (**6/1**) has combined with the assertiveness of the West (**9/4**) to put many a person with this Signature into executive offices. When sons or daughters with this Signature are expected to take over the family business, they will not only agree but step up and revamp the place! People with this Signature are practically born with the talent to be in the right spot at the right time.

Inventors, explorers, and pilots, among others, are at home in the North–West–Center and should not be held back in their younger years. If the Center of Gravity lies in the West, with both the Numbers **9** and **4**, a bearer's tendency to be a loner will increase, negatively impacting the collegiality and teamwork needed in an office setting. And the West's innate business sense could tip the scale toward ruthlessness, destroying any good results—it is a tightrope walk. A person with this Signature would not make a successful leader if he or she took care of every employee issue and lost sight of the long-term strategy in the process. The challenge in this case is finding the right balance between treating employees humanely and focusing on an efficient, competitive, long-term company strategy.

As always, the harmonious development of all talents depends on whether or not they were supported and allowed to unfold at an early age. If this did not happen, the child who bears this Signature in a family business might join the competition, either literally or metaphorically, and actually undermine the family business. In this instance, aggressive tendencies might come into play when it comes to coping with frustration. On the up-side, self-pity and resignation are far less likely with this Signature.

Genius and the abyss are rarely far apart; a split second can decide if a huge success is at hand or if a minor issue will destroy everything. With this Signature, the strength of the North (❻/❶) is important. Whether or not a brilliant invention is brought to fruition often depends on this Station because of the wise foresight it contributes. Its influence can be found within the Signature itself or in the successful collaboration with partners of the North. For this reason, bearers of this Signature are ideal for combining idea with implementation. Any negative tendencies caused by a surplus of energies of the West (❾/❹) will be balanced by the Center (0 / 5).

When remembering the unique energies of the Center—patience and the ability to recognize patterns—the danger of exaggeration is reduced and replaced by thoughtfulness and the ability to carefully weigh these considerations. Any danger zones can be discovered early and monitored. However, the invention or end result alone is never enough; the crucial point through the cycle of production is often the implementation phase. When West and North work in harmony, both invention and implementation are possible.

The North–West–Center Signature has only two missing Stations—the South (❼/❷) and the East (❽/❸). Ideally, co-workers or business partners whose strength lies in these Stations, or who bring their abilities to the table, are ideally suited for bearers of this Signature. Without this balance, both the business environment and the team dynamic could lack the necessary warmth and temperament required for success. Secretaries and assistants should definitely have some West (❾ or ❹) as well as some North (❻ or ❶), or they will find it difficult to be proactive in their work. Efficiency alone is not enough in this important function; there has to be a human side. Thanks to the Center, even without the East, this Signature radiates enough warmth and energy to have a firm grip on the business at hand.

The lacking temperament of the South can be balanced with red walls, tablecloths, candles, carpets, and so on, and people with this Signature should also always carry something red. A red bracelet alone would be effective. Additionally, the missing East could be balanced with the presence of the color green in clothing, at home, or on office furnishings. Houseplants are an excellent way to add green, too, as they are welcome everywhere and are easy to take care of. (Follow the moon calendar, and only water your plants on Cancer, Scorpio, and Pisces days. The success will speak for itself).

You should take the time to read up once more on your strengths and weaknesses in part 2. But don't look at all the possible combinations of individual Numbers with all the varying Stations of emphasis because the resulting mind game can be endless. Not only is this not the purpose, but it provides no significant help. It is enough for you to recognize yourself in these words and find inspiration to make more of your life. If you don't recognize yourself, then you might want to practice a bit with what you have read. Play with it in your thoughts to find out what is still hidden within you. Discover what you did not know until now, and enjoy the adventure!

North–South–Center

Convincing and charismatic– out into the world with the necessary vitality and power of the Center

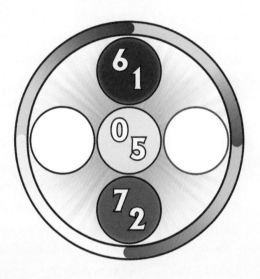

Yes, my dear Wilhelm, children are the closest thing
on earth to my heart. When I look at them
and see in these small beings the seeds of all the virtues,
all the powers that they will one day so urgently need;
when I glimpse future steadfastness and firmness of character
in their obstinacy and in their willfulness, good humor and ease
that will enable them to maneuver through the perils of the world,
everything so unspoiled, so of a piece!—
Then I repeat over and over the golden words of the teacher of mankind:
Unless you become as one of these!
—Johann Wolfgang von Goethe, *The Sorrows of Young Werther*
(*translated by Burton Pike*)

This Signature contains dates of birth with the Numbers

❻ and/or **❶**
❼ and/or **❷**
0 and/or **5**

The birthdates May 11, 1971; July 2, 2001; June 27, 1920; May 7, 1961; and February 5, 1966, are all examples of the North–Center–South Signature. Those of this signature are traveling on a different path, and sometimes on contradicting paths of the world and the soul. Education, life opportunities, willpower, and role models, when wisely applied or misguided, all play a big role and strongly imprint this child's soul.

Despite all our differences in character and life experience, there is a common thread: the shared treasure of the Code. The general direction of this Signature is toward public relations and the media, as bearers of the North–South–Center belong in the public eye no matter what the function or task, be it as a charismatic speaker or as a press secretary. The stronger your North is with **❻**s and **❶**s, the stronger its impact on you. And the more **❶**s in the Signature, the greater your visibility in public. If you don't quite see it that way but have the right Numbers, it may be the first hint that you should set many more goals in your life.

Let's take a look at the Center with the **0** and **5** (this Station truly represents the Center of life). It has all the characteristics to stay grounded and to resist the distractions of day-to-day life. Of course, education, habit, and unconscious action will affect your actual situation, but there is good news: despite all the difficulties you have encountered and have been delayed by on your path, you have the ability to overcome them. You say you don't feel this? Chances are you just haven't recognized the ability in yourself yet.

The **0** does have a small advantage over the **5**. If you have the **0** in your birthdate, you have a little of all the Birthday Wheel Numbers among your characteristics. That is why you recognize the luminous aura of the Center in the display of the Wheel. When the **0** wishes to extend its reasoning and emotional powers to the missing Stations, it will have fewer problems than others in doing so.

The vibrant South (**7**/**2**) provides this Signature with its highly ambitious energy. You not only have the ability to get things going in the media world but you are also an ideal candidate for positions requiring organizational savvy—film directing, management roles, serving on boards of directors, and so on. Given your missing West, you should definitely consider a partner with the **9** or **4** for handling business and other financial tasks. Your true abilities would not blossom fully if you had to deal with this type of work.

Your East (**8**/**3**) is also missing, and here, too, partners, colleagues, and team spirits can fill the void. Without the abilities of the East, you might be too coldly analytical when assessing a situation, inadvertently hurting others with your comments (this is the origin of the blunders that you sometimes make). The danger is even greater if you are an air sign (Gemini, Libra, or Aquarius), as air signs with this Signature are among those people who go their own way undeterred and free of self-doubt. They should be allowed to follow their destiny.

The fundamental task for you and all other Signatures is to maximize your gifts by filling your voids, which in your case are the West (**9**/**4**) and the East (**8**/**3**). Now would be a good time to reread the information about your personal Numbers in part 2. Take the time to look at the North, the Center, and the South as well; they are you. These are your talents! Allow this new awareness to flood your senses, and remember those times when everything felt right with the world. From now on, you might start a few things over in life—this time with the feeling that you are following your calling.

What does "filling the voids" mean for you? In part 2, reread the chapters on your missing Numbers to discern which powers, directions, and abilities are not strongly present in your Signature. This will help you gain more understanding at the same time; no one has to have *all* of the qualities. It is merely a matter of understanding.

The simplest way to fill the missing Cardinal Points is by incorporating the colors of these Stations—in your case, white and green. For example, you would benefit from more white and green in your wardrobe. Another good way to conquer the West is by practicing your manual skills in a hobby, or by strengthening your grip on the family finances—even if it is just checking the cash flow once a week.

Conversely, should you have a lot of Numbers in the North, you should avoid the colors blue and black, as they would intensify your Center of Gravity there. When the overemphasis occurs in the Center (if someone has the ⑤ twice, for example), you should avoid the color yellow. And with the South as the Center of Gravity, the color red should not move too much into the foreground. Repeat beneficial colors in your wardrobe, home, and food and when choosing which stones to carry with you. Give your fantasy free reign when it comes to kick-starting the motion of your personal Birthday Wheel and filling it with life.

East–West–Center

Artistic empathy with good business sense
balanced by a strong Center–
brilliant at times!

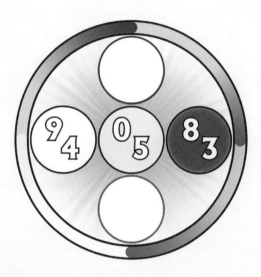

Take time to work—work is the price of success.
Take time to think—thoughts are the source of power.
Take time to play—play is the secret of perpetual youth.
Take time to be friendly—friendships give life a delicious flavor.
Take time to dream—dreams show you what is possible.
Take time to laugh—laughter is the music of the soul.
Take time to give—sharing brings joy to your heart.

—Icelandic proverb
(***translated by Thomas Poppe***)

This Signature contains dates of birth with the Numbers

8 and/or **3**
9 and/or **4**
0 and/or 5

The birthdates April 30, 1948; September 5, 1983; August 4, 1950; April 3, 2005; and May 8, 1994, are all examples of the East–West–Center Signature, which does not occur very often. The most frequent combinations are not possible here because the North (**6/1**) and the South (**7/2**) are missing; you were either born on the 3rd, 4th, 5th, 8th, or 30th. Only five months can be considered and only thirty-five of the years between 1900 and 2008.

These Numbers belong to extraordinary people who are well equipped for going it alone in life. (You remember meeting them; their presence filled the room.) Early on, they did not always know how to deal with this in a measured and healthy way, however. As a result, they need to distance themselves from people periodically. This need might be interpreted as arrogance (which it is at times), but in the course of their lives, they are often saved by the experience, energy, and empathy of the East (**8/3**).

Bearers of this Signature sometimes grapple with getting older. In order to distract themselves or make sure the problem of aging does not even rise to consciousness, they might choose much younger partners in their little flights from reality. Sometimes this works quite well without blocking true growth, which is the universal destiny. And the bearers of this Signature have a knack for connecting with young people, as their opinions tend to be current with the times, and make them popular conversationalists.

This Signature is persevering and precise; nothing is left to chance by being overly casual. The West (**9/4**) provides thorough thought, the Center (**0**/5) stands for reliability and faithfulness, and the East (**8/3**) brings amiability and sensitivity to the true needs of the moment. Isn't this a brilliant medley? However, there is the potential for a rude awakening if someone misuses these abilities. Instead of treating them as obligations, they should be treated as gifts.

A large number of brilliant musicians have this Signature. Generally, they are not only musical but have an above-average talent for playing instruments. It is a pure joy to listen to them, which is why it is especially important to encourage the innate musical talents and leanings of children with this Signature—even if they come from a nonmusical family. The sooner the better.

Developed talent does not just fall from the sky, but with the treasures that the East–West–Center gives its bearers, including the dazzling gem of musicality, they have a sizable head start over the rest of us.

This Signature also carries great talent for businesses of all types and should not be sacrificed to a false understanding of "being an artist." Good business sense and an intuitive grasp of soulful art *can* coexist. Bearers of this Signature have an innate talent for seemingly opposite things, and they combine talents that you would not expect in just one person. They compensate for the absent vibrancy of the South (❼/❷) with prowess.

If this is your Signature and you would like to bring your art to the public, you should look for partners who have the North (❻/❶) in their date of birth. However, you can handle business negotiations on your own. And when making public appearances, it would not hurt to wear black and red, as this provides security on all levels and allows you to conquer your missing Stations, the North and South.

If your Signature's Center of Gravity is in the West, you are more likely to become a banker, inventor, politician, mechanic, pilot, researcher, or explorer. If your Center is more prominently represented (maybe with a ❶ and a ❺), you are more suited for social service jobs where protective, observant people are needed. Conversely, a Center of Gravity in the East can result in a certain inner unrest because your awareness of unlived energies quickly surfaces. The danger is that resignation might become your prevailing mood, but this can be successfully countered by mustering the courage to live your own life.

In general people with this Signature possess not only an above average musicality, they are also especially gifted instrumentalists. Listening to them can be a pure joy.

Physicians, holistic healers, alternative healers, and psychologists are also heavily represented in the East because these people received the necessary capacity for empathy when they were born. (As an aside, physicians who are missing the compassionate East in their date of birth frequently become the proverbial "half-gods in white." They find their place on company boards instead of at patients' bedsides.)

All in all, live your talents and start immediately. No matter how old you are, get going! With this Signature, a terrific challenge awaits you. You can sing (or at least sing along) at any age. And you would not believe how many young entrepreneurs would be happy to receive good advice from you. It is immaterial how old you are. So you see, it is never too late, unless you believe it is, and accept and resign. And that's exactly what you are *not* going to do from now on, right?!

11. The Five Quads

North–East–South–Center

A multicolored palette of talents–
free of material constraints

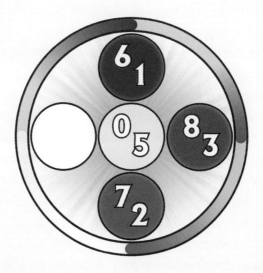

A human being is part of a whole, called by us the Universe,
a part limited in time and space.
He experiences himself, his thoughts and feelings,
as something separated from the rest
a kind of optical delusion of his consciousness.
This delusion is a kind of prison for us,
restricting us to our personal desires
and to affection for a few persons nearest us.
Our task must be to free ourselves from this prison
by widening our circles of compassion
to embrace all living creatures
and the whole of nature in its beauty.

—Albert Einstein

The dates of birth of this Signature contain only the Numbers

6 and/or **1**
8 and/or **3**
7 and/or **2**
0 and/or 5

The birthdates August 16, 2007; May 12, 1983; March 18, 1952; July 11, 1935; and December 13, 1983, are all examples of the North–East–South–Center Signature.

If one were to give each Signature a memorable title, then this Signature would be called "The Imaginative One." Its bearers do not *learn*, they instinctively *know*. Their keen interest, inordinate curiosity, profound gentleness, and passion for changes make those in this Signature so interesting. Their spiritual energy also gives them a "direct connection" to what is behind the scenes of all that is worldly. Superficial conversations are unlikely with these people, and you would be well advised to allow for a lot of time if you get into a conversation with them. Nothing bores this Signature more than mandatory invitations, bad movies, and small talk. The abilities of these people are so abundant, however, that they tend to have difficulty making decisions. Consequently, they are usually late bloomers and frequently have more than one professional phase over the course of a lifetime—so-called "life-stage careers"—as they progress in their development.

With so much talent at hand, one would almost prefer focusing on the few obstacles that pose as hindrances to this Signature rather than dwell on all the positive things that lie ahead. For example, everything in life, no matter what it is, needs careful attention if you would like to keep and preserve it. This applies to knowledge, opinions, and feelings as well. Being North–East–South–Center often comes with learned and drilled-in habits that you accepted in your younger years voluntarily. If you also accept the special challenge to free yourself, then the world is your oyster.

The missing West (**9**/**4**) could also have a grave impact if this is your Signature. Money is of little importance to you generally, so it might happen that your genius prevents you from being paid because you neglect to have a contract for work. One would think one learns through experience, but that is not necessarily true if you are the bearer of this Signature. Your overly generous trust can border on naiveté and place you in the same danger zone again and again.

Because of your unshakable belief in honest dealings, you must learn, much like a kindergartner learns the ABCs, the correct way to deal with the realities of the business world. It is just part of your spiritual makeup that you tend to find the rules of business life to be almost artificial and distressing, and thereby approach your business partners with mistrust. But you must learn how to balance that. Only by taking this step will you be able to live happily and in harmony—the way it is meant for you to live.

It is unfortunate that we have so few politicians with this Signature. (By now you probably know why.) For many, their trust is exploited early on in their careers, and they never make it to the very top. It is a paradox that their generosity—the very quality that could be most beneficial— becomes the obstacle to their success.

Whether you are a forester, athlete, actor, musician, healer, physician, geologist, singer, or painter, and whether you are male or female, anything is possible. If you sincerely want to have lasting success, then you need to look for a person whom you can trust unconditionally—but do not forget to have safeguards in place. Most likely, you will dislike this idea, because where there is trust, there is no need for safeguards, right? No! Your safeguards simply compensate for the missing West in your date of birth so you can feel at ease.

Reinforce your missing West with the color white wherever and whenever possible; wear white as part of your wardrobe. Your office should also have splashes of white since it is unlikely to be overly neat. Though you always find what you need, you are not about to waste any time with unimportant tasks like lining up pencils. Your likeable personality makes it easy for you to find a staff member who will happily organize for you—and that's OK; your talents lie in different area. There is no sense in frittering them away.

Another good way to conquer the West is to acquire a few manual skills by taking up a hobby that requires dexterity, like model building or other arts and crafts. There are many wonderful model kits available that are easy enough for anyone to assemble and look beautiful on display. Another way to conquer the West is to focus on the family finances by reviewing your weekly, monthly, and/or yearly spending. All of this sharpens the senses needed to liberate the special energies of the West.

When your life comes to an end, future generations will enjoy the bounty of good that will be your legacy. And with the start of the new millennium, the North–East–South–Center Signature is appearing much more often—a blessing for us all.

East–South–West–Center

With heart and mind all paths are open– including the quiet ones

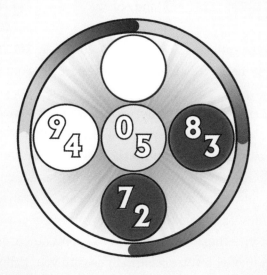

There is a piece of paradise in each smile,
In each good word, in the affection that you give away.
God put his love into your hands,
Like a key to paradise.

—Phil Bosmans
(translated by Thomas Poppe)

The dates of birth of this Signature contain only the Numbers

⑧ and/or ❸
❼ and/or ②
❾ and/or ❹
⓪ and/or ⑤

The birthdates September 8, 1975; April 23, 2005; May 28, 1994; March 25, 1942; and July 9, 1958, are all examples of the East–South–West–Center Signature.

Certain Signatures are virtually perfect when it comes to furnishing a treasure trove of talents and special abilities. If this is your Signature, it would be advantageous now to quickly review your Numbers again in part 2—East (❽/❸), South (❼/②), West (❾/❹), and Center(⓪/⑤). You will clearly recognize that a special life plan can be drawn with all these colors and abilities—a life that offers a very promising, multicolored scenario. You must give these abilities room to express their qualities in your life, however, so that who you become aligns with your calling.

There are people who use a few of their Numbers to do a lot with their life; they turn coal into diamonds. Others make little use of their given talents. Although inactivity is hardly ever a problem with this Signature, there could still be brief periods when certain energies seem to be wasted. This is because the talents at play here prefer to work behind the scenes. If you have this Signature, it might be hard sometimes to tell if you avoid the limelight on purpose, or if you just happen to be in the background.

As soon as you have reached your goal, you tend to move on to the next thing without looking back or taking a break to enjoy the fruits of your labor. Your journey itself is your destination. Perhaps you are actually chasing a goal that is invisible to those around you; people with this Signature are often secretive. There is, however, no reason for secrecy since they frequently have much greater abilities than they admit to themselves. This hesitancy may be rooted in shyness and anxiety dating back to their childhood. Despite your abundant talents as a bearer of the East,

South, West, and Center, you have a tendency to ruminate and to doubt yourself. "I will never manage that." "This is too expensive." "It takes too long." "What will others say?" "I don't want to move so far away." The list is potentially endless. If you find yourself trapped by these worries, a few minutes of meditation might do the trick. Having the North's colors— black and blue—in your wardrobe would also be very helpful, as these colors provide the necessary counterbalance to slow you down and calm your thoughts.

People whose Signature contains both the South (❼/❷) and the East (❽/❸) are generally well liked. They are also excellent with finances and detailed planning as a result of the West (❾/❹). With the Center (0 / 5) present as well, they are good sports and are nearly always sensible. This is a fortunate quality because, as the saying goes, "Two hearts often beat in one chest," requiring this person to balance the rational, sometimes too-cold calculations of the West with the romantic thoughts of the East.

The missing North (❻/❶) could occasionally be problematic for you, as the four Cardinal Points of your Signature create a deep thirst for knowledge. Since the pure energy of the North needs to be discovered and harnessed (a lifetime task for this Signature), the ability to set priorities can be impaired. Many people have no idea about the variety of experiences and possibilities available in life; they know only what is directly in front of their faces. With this Signature, the opposite holds true. These people are interested in so many things in life that they can sometimes feel crushed by an infinite expanse of choices.

If you are a bearer of this Signature, there is hardly anything that you are not capable of doing. However, the absence of the North (❻/❶) sometimes prevents you from profound access to certain themes in your life. You may despair as you sense that there are countless alternatives involved in taking any next step. The good news is that you merely lack the ability to make a decision because the decision that would put everything back on track is not easily available to you. That is also the reason why you do things that other people would never think of doing; this can be a positive thing. It is what makes this Signature brilliant and unique.

There are many people who love the color black and use it to set themselves apart. Some of these people are compensating, often unconsciously, for what is missing in their Signature. Given your Stations, working with the colors black and blue would be a big step forward. These colors are calming, slowing you down, and encouraging meditation while providing you with the necessary insight for making sound decisions.

The missing North also means that the negative aspects of this Station are not present. Hence, people with this Signature rarely succumb to the fanaticism or nervous tension from which so many suffer today. People with this Signature are also not quick to anger and are rarely considered a detriment to their community.

On your path to wholeness, create additional balance by paying attention to the position of your Center of Gravity, which is based on the last number of your birth year and the Station where you have the most Units; it can awaken your spirits and sharpen your insight. Assuming the East is your Center of Gravity (for example, if you were born in 19❽❸), the slow pace of learning to play an instrument might be the right approach for you. With it, you will come to understand the need to settle down and concentrate on your goal. Alternately, there are many people with this Signature who intuitively fill their voids by acquiring a profession with Numbers they do not have. Anything is possible with this Signature.

North–South–West–Center

A sharp mind with passion and genius–
for a better world

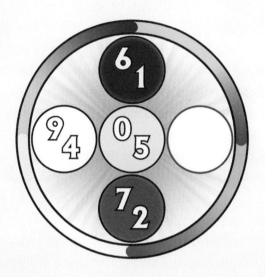

May you always have work for your hands to do.
May your pockets hold always a coin or two.
May the sun shine bright on your windowpane.
May the rainbow be certain to follow each rain.
May the hand of a friend always be near you.
And may God fill your heart with gladness to cheer you.
—Irish travel blessing

The dates of birth of this Signature contain only the Numbers

6 and/or **1**
7 and/or **2**
9 and/or **4**
0 and/or **5**

The birthdates January 5, 1992; May 10, 1974; July 16, 1995; September 7, 1965; and April 17, 2005, are all examples of the North–South–West–Center Signature, which has a wealth of Numbers.

When a person with this Signature makes an appearance, everyone is happy. And "making an appearance" is indeed the correct phrase, because these people are not just present; when they enter a room, they *appear*. All are impressed by their charisma, and they are accustomed to being the center of attention. As a result, they cannot take the backseat when another charismatic person is present. But this should not be construed as a sign of chronic jealousy. On the contrary, these people merely want to participate in everything that happens around them. They have abilities that others can only dream about and can master virtually any situation. They look for loopholes and solutions, rarely lack ideas, and are always willing to try the untried. And in addition to having manual skills as well as the intelligence to tackle the task at hand, they can do both under pressure.

You say you have this Signature but do not recognize yourself? Then someone must have done a good job of tying up your talents and energies. We cannot encourage you enough to begin unearthing this treasure now. It is never too late.

Living with bearers of this Signature on a daily basis is not always easy. Others find their constant solicitousness and inordinate curiosity to be too much (they rarely miss anything). And when those around them become aware of their X-ray vision, it can consciously or unconsciously be considered an intrusion. However, the people of this Signature merely want to offer their help so that others do not repeat their mistakes. They just have to keep in mind that people are not "making a mistake" but are gathering the life experience needed for their own for self-confidence and stability. One of this Signature's life tasks is learning to watch calmly when others, especially children, make mistakes in the process of gathering these life experiences.

Actors and politicians, as well as brilliant musicians, frequently have this Signature. They are able to assert themselves, are listened to, and have a knack for business. And what they do not know, they simply learn. Only the missing East (❽/❸) can be a source of pain at times. Since the emotional life is at home in the East, the emptiness there does not diminish the chances of a materially successful professional life. It is amazing, however, to watch what the partners of this Signature have to put up with at times. Since the bearers of this Signature are otherwise likeable and honest, often a blind eye is turned on certain traits as long as the "impertinence" does not become a permanent fixture.

We have all seen and experienced when professional practices fall by the wayside, like calling in sick to work on the day of the big presentation. This type of behavior is totally agitating to people of this Signature, and depending upon his or her mood that day, he or she might even become slightly hysterical. If you, like this Signature, are accustomed to having a solution at hand for everything, this kind of distressed response is bound to happen once in a while. (And with a bit of luck, the rest of us will be far enough away to avoid bearing the brunt of such an outburst.) The people of this Signature benefit greatly from long walks and from time spent in nature.

Children with this Signature, as well as all children whose East is missing, should never be left alone, especially not without their knowledge. Children of this Signature tend to be sympathetic to everything and need the assurance of trust; that is why it is also important to never lie to them— even little white lies. This point is true for all children, who still have very sensitive antennae. As adults, we tune out many signals or block them so that we can no longer hear them. Children sense this weakness and appreciate the strength and the straightforwardness of the truth. They learn to handle it in a positive way whether they like what they are hearing or not.

Lies of all types result in much anger, evaporate trust, and make a lot of work for a partnership.

If this is your Signature but you have not fulfilled your dreams by living the life that will make you happy, then simply start today. You are never too old to make a fresh start. The world is waiting for you.

North–East–West–Center

Conquering the world from a balanced center–
willing, ready, and able

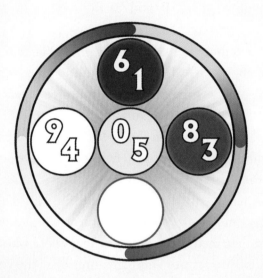

The greatest and noblest pleasure
Which men can have in this world
Is to discover new truths;
And the next is to shake off old prejudice
                    —Frederick II of Prussia,
                    known as Frederick the Great

The dates of birth of this Signature contain only the Numbers

6 and/or **1**
8 and/or **3**
9 and/or **4**
0 and/or 5

The birthdates September 8, 1951; June 13, 1995; March 5, 1991; March 9, 1968; and November 13, 1945, are all examples of the North–East–West–Center Signature—a Signature that brings its bearer a great deal of joy.

The greater the variety in the Numbers of a person's Signature and the more widespread the Numbers in the Birthday Wheel, the more difficult it is to describe the Number treasure. These people have so many abilities that all that we can say is, "Terrific!"

Anyone who has spent a lot of time working with the Code is accustomed to seeing people with missing Stations having to do repairs. They sometimes appreciate their successes more than those who were born with a substantial Number treasure. This Signature's one little void in the Birthday Wheel is not that noticeable, so it can get ignored. Should this be your Signature, then you surely know from personal experience what this means. However, the good news is that even the tiniest void can be filled to everyone's advantage.

Let's assume that, despite having this terrific Signature, you continue to have difficulties reaching certain goals. In that case, we would like to recommend the simplest, most effective technique for you: bring more red into your life. The missing South (**7**/**2**) makes the bearer think they frequently get shortchanged. Such a feeling could lead to true heartache and shouldn't be lightly dismissed as a passing weakness. If this rings a bell with you, you should work on it when it occurs. It can feel miserable if you believe you are not being taken seriously or do not count, even if the actual facts do not support that belief. Use more red in your life—in your wardrobe, home, and workplace. This will keep that feeling at bay. Keep an eye on your personal biorhythms as well. We all run the danger of falling into such traps, especially in the fourteen-day cycles on the weekday of our birth. (You can read more about biorhythms in our book *Moon Time*.)

The bearers of this Signature have been handsomely blessed with emotions, so much so that they sometimes do not know what to do with them all. They cannot bear cheating and tend to remember those incidents for their entire life. For them "cheating" is a broad term for a variety of occasions. After all, it is cheating if trust is betrayed or if someone is abandoned. It might be helpful for people with this Signature to concentrate more on their own goals. If they wait until others catch up, they end up becoming exasperated; not everyone has the same prerequisites. Their high standards are exhausting for other people, sometimes unbearably so. Being with a person who is a perfectionist in many areas of life requires an especially patient personality.

If this is your Signature, you are assured success. It does not matter if you sell cars or are a famous actor; whether you fight for minorities or are a top athlete, inventor, or politician. You are well equipped for all of these, and once you have made a decision, you will succeed. If you feel discontent, it generally does not stem from feeling incapable but from a lingering sense that "it could have been better." You need to remember that everyone has different gifts and talents. Be a little more lenient. Cut yourself and those around you some slack. Teamwork can be one of your strengths, but not necessarily. For those times when teamwork is necessary, you should find colleagues who have the South (❼/❷) as part of their Signature.

The South alone will not be enough, of course. The necessary abilities for the tasks at hand also need to be brought along. In this instance, a person's Zodiac sign can play a role. Fire signs (Aries, Leo, and Sagittarius) sometimes do not notice the missing South in their Signature because the energies of their Zodiac sign have a balancing effect.

Since you are the life of the party for all festivities, you are always a welcome guest at performances and other get-togethers. Use these opportunities to replenish your South and you will rediscover the feeling that you have missed for so long—the sense that you belong and are important.

And once the party is over, be careful not to fall back into the black hole of self-doubt. You have high standards and would rather be alone than compromise your principles. That is fine. You are warmhearted, honest, and have a sharp mind. You are entitled to your ambitions.

It would be best to use the color red as medicine in your life on a permanent basis. Red can help you master all challenges while rounding out your talents along your unique path. The happier you are, the happier we'll all be, too.

North–East–South–West

All roads are open– dreams can become reality

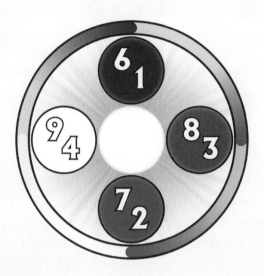

As long as we have dreams, we live.
As long as we live, dreams give us hope.
As long as there is hope, we are not afraid of the future.
The future lies in our hands.
Let's not just dream it, but live it.

—Petra Heierhoff
(translated by Thomas Poppe)

The dates of birth of this Signature contain only the Numbers

6 and/or **1**
8 and/or **3**
7 and/or **2**
9 and/or **4**

The birthdates July 8, 1969; September 12, 1988; April 8, 1976; June 3, 1992; and February 13, 1994, are all examples of the North–East–South–West Signature, or the "Ring Signature," as it is also known.

All four of the Cardinal Points adorn your Signature, and that is a wonderful thing! You are ideally equipped to reach every imaginable goal in life. From the bottom of our hearts, we hope that you perceive the value in this gift. Hopefully, you have already actualized it. Bearers of this Signature ponder, test, tinker, and think—and then are ready to go. They achieve brilliant things without much ado and take for granted what others see as an unattainable goal. It is very pleasant to work with people who have a strong self-confidence built on sincerity and substance, and you have the ideal prerequisites to lay such a foundation.

It is a good thing for everyone that you exist. Your Signature will casually take its time in the twenty-first century and shine with terrific inventions, songs, publications, literary themes, new releases, and improvements of every imaginable thing. Which professions are suitable for this Signature? There is no need to list them. You can do anything that you set your mind to.

Despite so much good news, there is one little fly in the ointment: "want" is a key word here. "Wanting" is the setback with you. The high standards you set for yourself and others can occasionally delay a decision for or against a certain path. Those around you do not always appreciate the apparent slowdown, because it taxes their patience. And you can suddenly become very angry because others' admonishments interrupt your "constructive dreaming." In rare instances, your anger can change to downright stubbornness and obstinacy, or it may even turn into false pride.

Generally, bearers of this Signature have a likable disposition, which makes them pleasant contemporaries. They are anything but spoilsports, having fun but still paying enough attention to the successful completion of the important things in life. This is a rare combination in this day and age. As a bearer, you may spend a few days daydreaming before you make your first move. It may appear to others that nothing is happening during these days, but that is only the outward appearance. In reality, you have been thinking long and hard, and you'll only take action after all the intricacies of the task at hand have been thought through.

It is here that we encounter a small problem that this Signature occasionally has to battle, especially among the children with this combination of Stations in this day and age. The adage "Good wine takes time" does not really fit in the Computer Age. However, that does not change its validity. And no one knows that better than a child born with this Signature.

As a bearer, you have been showered with so much abundance that you may not appreciate your many talents, or it may be that you have not completely actualized your talents, failing to transform them into lively actions. You often do not know what it is like to be unable to do something. Normally, brilliant people are long dead before they are truly appreciated, but not in your case. You assert yourself during your lifetime and you are heard. It takes time, but you will succeed. Never fail to take the time you need!

No other Signature is as misunderstood as this one. Why? Because you work quietly and appear only when you have something worthwhile to say. Of course, you do not work quietly all of the time, but in the beginning, your work takes place in the background. It is not your style to shout things from the rooftops in the initial phases, which is probably due to your missing Center (**0** / **5**).

You are not the only one with whom the Center void causes feelings of discontent. Normally, there is no outwardly visible reason for this, but you may see it differently. You often feel misunderstood and need affection from home; a strong Center creates that feeling of a nurturing environment. Using the color yellow in your daily life would quickly bring relief—a safe harbor—and fill the void. Having a lot of yellow in your wardrobe and eating yellow food are additional ways to do this. Sometimes it also helps to eat something sweet, as this taste is connected to the color yellow (but make sure that it is an organic product!).

Spending considerable time in nature is beneficial as well. Walk, gather mushrooms, photograph flowers—do whatever calms the spirit. Any activity that is connected to the earth would literally ground you emotionally and re-establish your Center. You could also have lots of flowers in your home, or keep a small herb garden on your balcony or windowsill. The important thing is that the presence of nature compensates for the empty Center.

We would all be happy if we were able to awaken our understanding of the dreaming nature of this Signature. And now you know why this is part of your life. It is a step on your path to happiness.

12

All the Cardinal Points on the Birthday Wheel

North–East–South–West–Center

All paths are open

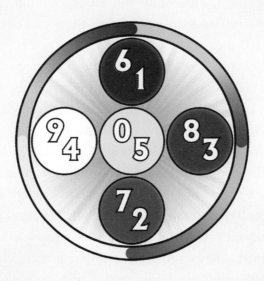

*We are adequately equipped
for all our genuine earthly needs
if we will trust our senses,
and develop them in such a way
that they continue to prove worthy of our confidence.*
—Johann Wolfgang von Goethe

This Signature contains dates of birth with all the Numbers

6 and/or **1**
8 and/or **3**
7 and/or **2**
9 and/or **4**
0 and/or **5**

The birthdates May 21, 1998; October 17, 1985; October 23, 1949; December 8, 1990; and May 19, 1978, are all examples of the rare Signature in which all Cardinal Points are present.

One would almost say that you have won the lottery with this Signature! Hardly anything is difficult for you. However, if difficulty does occur, any weakness that surfaces does not reflect the actual talents with which you were born. It comes instead as a result of later events.

This wealth of Numbers provides bearers of this Signature with ample choices when deciding on a profession. In their younger years, this overwhelming abundance of interests can lead to an inner logjam of choices. Late bloomers are not uncommon in this Signature.

It would be best to put financial considerations on the back burner and choose what brings you the greatest joy. You will do a good job, whether you take over a business or build it from scratch, design houses or write books. Since not all of your talents are distributed in equal proportions, we suggest that you trust your instincts. And if your instincts remain muddled and chaotic, you should gather as many different experiences as possible. Your personal calling will eventually crystallize in its own good time.

The best way to make your decision is to first consider that the last Number in your date of birth—your year of birth—has the strongest influence. For example, if you were born in 1962, the **2** is the most dominant. Take a closer look at the professions in the table on page 263 and open yourself up to the options there. If you were born in 1963, the East's **3** is stronger, so musical talent and the ability to heal move into the forefront.

Second, with this special Signature, only one Station can have double Numbers, which means that it is virtually impossible to form a Center of Gravity or become unbalanced in any area. Whatever you choose, any choice will give you an equal chance to find your calling and be successful at it.

You probably remember from your school years those children who had everything land in their lap without much effort. We are not referring to the overachievers who keep everything to themselves and do not know the meaning of teamwork, eventually becoming tyrants and subservient yes-men. No, we are referring to those children who never cram but always seem to pass somehow, albeit sometimes by the skin of their teeth. These are the children of this rare Signature, and therein lies one of their problems. Since everything comes to them easily, they often sit around bored and do not pay attention to anything. They miss opportunities and are labeled as troublemakers or "problem children." Fortunately, this is usually only a passing phase in their lives, and their talents are sufficient to make up for what they missed.

In another scenario, these children and teens still never make an effort but get excellent grades regardless. If there is ever a time when they need to persevere and cram, however, they struggle because they lack experience with tedious, everyday life. Then, when special expertise needs to be acquired later in life and a fully booked calendar puts pressure on them, they may not know how to juggle everything at once. This is one of the reasons they may fall by the wayside when the going gets tough. A lot depends on the child's upbringing, talents notwithstanding, and moderation is not one of their inborn gifts. There is definitely a risk that their energy will disipate over the long term.

Some days, no one knows why things go haywire or why nothing is moving (see the section "The Power of the Actual Date" in part 4), and this is usually connected to the Numbers of that calendar date. Many Signature bearers can practice utilizing the favorable energies of the actual date or can learn to deal wisely with the unfavorable energies. This does not necessarily apply to this Signature since it has everything to begin with! For example, bearers of a Signature without a South (**7**/**2**) in their birthday could have used the year 20 **0** **7** to their advantage because the entire year provided complementing impulses. However, bearers of Signatures with the Center of Gravity in the South or with an excessive South may have been ill more frequently than usual in 2007.

"Heavy is the head that wears the crown"—a proverb that applies especially to this last Signature. We are happy for anyone who was born with these Numbers. May the biggest problem in your life be too many opportunities! And may you see and understand a broad perspective while keeping your eye on the right path.

◆　　◆　　◆　　◆　　◆

If you have read all the preceding pages, by the time you have reached this point, you know that each Signature—each person—has the opportunity to make the best of his or her life. This is assuming, of course, that we completely unpack our treasure chests and use our bounty out of love for ourselves and in gratitude for free will—a gift to all of us.

We hope that we have disclosed many a useful secret, as we want to bring you the joy of shaping your own future. Always trust your instincts. And the Code will provide good support and help along the way.

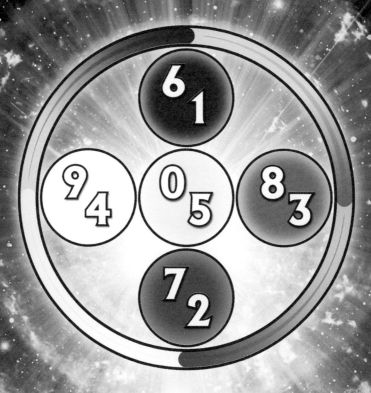

Part 4

The Code in Practice

13

The Signatures in Everyday Life

In part 1 of this book, we described the basics of the Code and the Birthday Wheel. In part 2, we brought to life the individual Cardinal Points of the Birthday Wheel so that you might get an idea of the gems in your personal treasure of Numbers. Part 3 showed the individual Signatures, and the unique gifts and challenges for each one. Now, in part 4, we will describe some larger workings of the Code, the Code in everyday life, and how the Code is used in healing.

The descriptions of the Signatures in part 3 were meant to provide you with an overview of the interplay of the Cardinal Points in each individual case. You got to know the dynamics of your personal Signature and those of other Signatures, whose bearers could be family members, business associates, or people you would like to support or know more about. It could also be a person you do not get along with, possibly because all attempts to reach them have failed to date. Now their Signature provides insight into how to connect with them.

The thirty-one Signatures on the Birthday Wheel demonstrate the liveliness and the dynamics of the Code, and as you can see, there are clearly defined tasks that are reflected in the individual Numbers of one's personal Code. Occasionally, this may have felt like trying to catch smoke with your bare hands, but we're confident that it was worthwhile. How successful we were is now up to you to decide.

Just as one gradually becomes familiar with a new instrument or a tool, he or she inevitably encounters one or another problem during the training stages. But that is what manuals are for, are they not? At this point, however, there is a possibility that after reading about your personal Signature, you may have gotten the impression that your own Code—its Numbers and Signature—characterize and bind you, as if you were genetically predisposed to certain things. There is also the possibility that you recognized certain "types" of people in the other Signatures to whom you attribute, in the worst case, unchangeable, fateful characteristics. If this is the case, you run the risk of arbitrarily labeling yourself and others, or hiding behind predetermined assumptions, thus hampering the development of personal responsibility and free will. Do not fall prey to these dangerous false impressions about the Signatures. The knowledge of the Code should be regarded as life-enhancing information that is meant to be playfully assimilated into your everyday affairs at your own pace.

We hope that your Signature makes for interesting reading—like an honest and well-meaning short story written about you by a good friend. Surely, there will be quite a few "aha" moments, and a lot of smiling and laughing when reading the story with others and exchanging thoughts. And many a finger might be pointed with the exclamation, "See, isn't this what I've been saying all along?" Or, "Finally! Now you have it in black and white." Or even, "Well, no wonder, with those Numbers!" These cheerful, revelatory moments of recognition are common when learning about the Code—and one reason why we wrote this book.

Take a look at the cover of the book again, and contemplate the ring around the Wheel and the rays that emanate from its Center. Here, you can see the movement of a dynamic spiral—a work of art in motion, developing as it matures. If you are unhappy with your development but don't know why, this book can show you your unique path that leads to happiness.

The secret is knowing yourself and what makes you thrive. The eagle spirit among men belongs in the fresh, thin air of the mountains, not in an air-conditioned office; whereas the bean counter, happily buried between financial ledgers, would gasp for breath at alpine heights. Much of the world's misfortunes come from lacking the courage and keen insight to follow our own individual paths—the path the angels marked for us. Without at least a spark of genuine faith, no one is likely to find true meaning and the right life path. Anyone who is kind and compassionate can despair when reading the morning paper, and only genuine faith can help. It is the first step on the journey to knowledge.

The Dynamic Aspects of the Birthday Wheel

This book poses four questions to you:

- ◆ What are my Numbers?
- ◆ What do my Numbers signify?
- ◆ Which Numbers am I missing?
- ◆ What can I do now?

Once you know your Numbers and those you are missing, you have several possibilities available to you. One option is to live your Numbers to the limit and try out all possibilities of your treasure. Another possibility is to look for a way to compensate for your missing Numbers and to explore areas in the map of your soul. These choices enrich your palette with the missing colors, and in return, you gain a rainbow, the wholeness of the spirit.

There are always several other possibilities. You may feel that there is something missing because you have a void in your Birthday Wheel that is affecting your happiness. Or maybe you have the Numbers and aren't living them because you forgot how, someone drove them out of you, or you were afraid. Having many Numbers that lie fallow is sometimes worse than having merely a few Numbers that are allowed to develop. The palette of possibilities for opening up, maturing, and becoming whole has colors that are as infinite as the number of ways to resist these tasks and adventures. The choice is yours!

Exercising free will contributes to the dynamic, constant movement of the Birthday Wheel and, depending on your choices, influences how you transform your Signature into a work of art in motion. We also would like to mention three other essential factors that lend additional dynamics, momentum, and character to the Numbers and their distribution on the Wheel.

First Dynamic Aspect: Weigh the Units

In part 1, we discussed the Units, which are the first dynamic aspect of your personal Code. How many Units did you count in each of your Cardinal Points?

By now, you know that the sum of the Units in any Cardinal Point is simply the sum of its numerical values. You also know that any Cardinal Point with more than ten Units can result in extreme overdevelopment, which can be either positive or negative. To give you a few examples, if you were born on May 9, 1979, you have two ❾s in the West. This means you have eighteen Units of the energies inherent in this Station. Having the Number ❾ once on your Wheel generally means that you have good business sense. Two ❾s on the Wheel, however, can turn this financial savvy into egotism and willfulness. Wise business foresight, in other words, has the potential to become miserliness and a desperate clinging to worldly goods and relationships.

Perhaps you were born on May 3, 1988. This means you have nineteen Units in your East. The East is the home of deep empathy, but if you have that many Units of this special energy, your empathy can strengthen to the point that you can become too considerate, neglecting your own needs. After a while, the other extreme can set in, and you end up opposing your own exploitation to the point of becoming egotistical (often to the surprise of those who know you). The East's big talent—its valuable treasure—is then squandered, and the great empathy of its bearers withdraws into a shell. They become outwardly reserved and cool as empathy and compassion are locked away in a safe of apparent heartlessness. This lasts until empathy is revived with the help of insight and the slow process of learning moderation. For those the with East in their Stations, "Love your neighbor as you love yourself" means striking a sensible balance between giving and taking. If you are born with more than ten Units in any Cardinal Point, one of your life tasks consists of learning to manage the danger of excess.

Consequently, it is clear that it would not be such a good idea to force the selection of a round number for a birthdate when scheduling a Caesarean section, a common form of delivery today. The child is not only endowed with double or triple energy in a Cardinal Point on the Wheel (with the danger of a subsequent overdevelopment), but he or she is saddled with special challenges and expectations at the same time. It is best to look at any date as a special offering, whatever the resulting Signature may be.

Second Dynamic Aspect: Consider the Difference between the Numbers of a Station

The second dynamic aspect of the Birthday Wheel rests upon the fine difference between the two Numbers found in each Cardinal Point. Let's use several dates of birth and draw a Birthday Wheel sketch to demonstrate this point.

Looking at the sketches on the next page, you can see immediately that all four birthdates form the same Signature—North–East–Center (see also page 165).

The 0 is weighed differently than the 5 in a birthdate, since the 0 provides direct access to all Stations and the 5 develops a keen sense for nature in general. (You can read about these differences in part 2 and in previous chapters.) Similarly, the Numbers 1 through 5 carry masculine energy, whereas the Numbers 6 to 0 carry feminine energy (as mentioned in part 1). Keep these subtle differences in mind with these sketches and whenever you work with the Code.

As another example, although the dates of birth May 1, 1966, and May 10, 1955, both have the North–Center Signature, different characters will form from the same Signature to reveal varying treasure chests for each

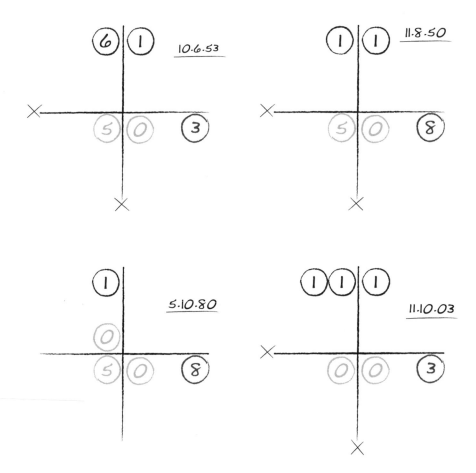

bearer. However, the general talent setup is the same. The formation of different Centers of Gravity in a Signature stands out more when only two or three Stations are occupied with the four to six possible Numbers. The Singles are clear-cut in their distribution of energies (see page 89), and the Signatures with four and all five Stations also allow for more even distribution (see page 189 and page 209). When contemplating the Signatures, you should add these differences to your experiences with them.

Third Dynamic Aspect: Find the Center of Gravity
The third aspect that provides extra momentum to each Signature lies in which Numbers have the most emphasis in your Signature. As an example,

let's pick four more dates of birth with the exact same Number distribution and Signature.

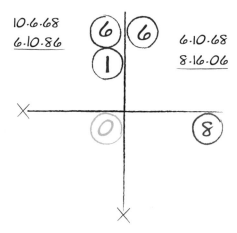

You can see from the drawing above that the Number distribution we've chosen leads to an overemphasis in the North, with two ❻s giving us twelve Units (more than ten Units). However, a strong emphasis in a Cardinal Point does not necessarily equate to an overweighing in that Station. For example, in the birthdate June 10, 1986, the North, where the energy of researchers is at home, is heavily emphasized because of the ❻ in the birth year. Yet when we consider another birthdate, say June 10, 2008, the center of power shifts; the ❻ is coming from the month, not the year, and we have an ❽ for the year. As a result of the ❽'s presence, the child will be more prone to emotion, and this will have a bearing on the child's future and career path (musicality, healing abilities). It should also be pointed out that both of the people above are Cancers, so the special energies of that Zodiac sign, like heightened sensitivity, also come into play here.

In general, you can assume that a ❻ from the day of birth will have a lesser impact than a ❻ from the birth year. The birth year has the greater weight, and its Cardinal Point should be developed and lived, as it carries more energy and useful powers than the other Numbers. Someone born on January 2❻, 1978, who does not integrate the unique, visionary energy of the ❻ into his or her life plan will be less affected by the missing Number than a person who was born on March 24, 197❻. But keep this in mind: having a ❻ in your day of birth that is lovingly developed and supported is, all things considered, more valuable than having a dried-up, blocked ❻ in one's year of birth. You can observe again and again that a Signature is a moving work of art that cannot be pinned down.

By the way, the formation of the Center of Gravity and the weight of the birth year are also the reasons why a milestone birthday—like one's 50th, 70th, or even 100th birthday—have always warranted special celebrations. Birthdays with a milestone number make the birthday child conscious of having their "very own year," reinforcing its importance over a lifetime.

These examples are not meant to confuse you (though this is common when you first start working with the Birthday Wheel). Over time, you will find that your ability to interpret any Signature on the Birthday Wheel increases with your understanding of each particular person. The subtleties and the multitude of aspects involved with anyone's personal Code reveals the Birthday Wheel and its many fascinating facets. The proof is in the pudding!

How can you best cultivate the life opportunities afforded to you on the Birthday Wheel? Even if you are approaching eighty, ninety, or one hundred years, you always have the ability to start fresh. To insist otherwise is only ingrained laziness of the soul and the destructive habit of justification. Naturally, this book cannot create heaven on earth for you overnight, especially if one has lived forty, fifty, or even sixty years against his or her own instincts. But regardless of where you are in life, a short daily meditation on the question "What would happen if I ...?" can help. Simply imagining what might happen if you encourage the talents and energies inherent in your Numbers will no doubt bring results. You will find the special switch to illuminate the rooms within your soul; it is never too late.

◆ ◆ ◆ ◆ ◆

The information we just presented can be used much like a nutritional guide. Let's assume you are thin, healthy, fit, and happy. Why in the world would you need nutritional advice? At best, it would make you aware that you are doing everything right and encourage you to continue, perhaps with even more discipline. On the other hand, you may not be happy, and you may have tried everything without long-term success. This yo-yo effect is driving you to desperation as you continue to fall into the same trap. Do you give in to your ravenous appetite, so to speak? Whatever the case, let this guide help you along a different path—one that you feel is intuitively right and to which your heart and mind say yes. Working with the Code might be the first step on a long journey. You might suddenly communicate better with your children because you now understand each other, which will inevitably lead to a better relationship.

We have shown you the voids that need filling, where and when you have Numbers missing, and which spaces need to be conquered as part of your birthright. Even if you are generally happy, this information can help you to better understand your partner, your children, and your contemporaries. Hidden in the Numbers and their effect are two proverbs, "Birds of a feather flock together" and "Opposites attract." This is not a contradiction in terms, even though it would be difficult for things to appear more oppositional.

Oppositional Signatures can complement each other beautifully and to the benefit of all. For example, this type of pairing happens when a lenient and "client-friendly" person of the East opens a business and takes on a partner who has the West in his Signature, ensuring that the business operates in the black. Woe, if after years of harmonious cooperation, one Signature tries to emulate the other Signature! This could happen in a small business if the "soul of the bookkeeping department," who has a ❾ or ❹, decides to take on customer service without having Numbers in the East or a ⓿. We are not saying that this type of endeavor will necessarily fail, but there is sure to be some sort of upheaval.

Similar Signatures can also harmonize beautifully—in synch, for the greater good. However, this does involve the risk of mutually reinforcing each other to stand still; you could complement each other's fears and maintain the status quo instead of encouraging each other to reach for new horizons. This is not a problem as long as both of you love where you are and want to remain there. The problem arises when one person breaks free after years of stalemate, and the one left behind finds it difficult to have empathy for the person who moved on.

◆   ◆   ◆   ◆   ◆

What if you do not recognize yourself in your Signature? Do not be fooled if the description does not match your present self-awareness; there are many ways to successfully resolve contradictions. For instance, let's assume that someone has become a mathematical genius or the successful founder of a software company without having the West's ❾ or ❹. Or someone has become a great musician, despite the lack of an ❽ or ❸ in his date of birth. Or another person has dedicated herself to running a successful organic farm without having a ⓪ or ⑤ in her date of birth.

We could give many more examples for such seeming contradictions. Very often, these are people who were afraid to relinquish control at an early age, and they made up for the missing Stations in their choice of profession (because after all, they are at home and in control of their own Cardinal Points). Or such seemingly contradictory people started to fill the voids in their Birthday Wheel early in life, as children instinctively do. In some cases, they might have had external influences—parents, media, teachers, and contemporaries—who led them to develop the talents of their missing Numbers. Having a ⓪ in one's Signature is also a strong component to successfully dealing with one's missing Numbers (see page 73).

When you look closely, you will often find that these "contradictory" people make a hobby of their Numbers instead of living them out in day-to-day life. Or perhaps a company president, who does not have the ❾ or ❹ in his date of birth but does have the ❽ or ❸, rises up to be a very humane boss, providing ample benefits for his employees, such as free company day care. At the same time, he makes up for the lack of the ❾ and the ❹ by having a highly efficient staff with these Numbers. Or take the case of the diehard workaholic with a Center of Gravity in the West (❾/❹) who does not make it home before 10 PM—perhaps he opens up with regular walks in the woods, by growing plants on his balcony, and through love of specific herbs.

In most cases, the seeming contradiction between self-image and the description of one's Signature dissolves when looking closely with an informed, open mind.

The Signature of Children

People often ask us how they should approach the varying Signatures of their children, and we have a few very important recommendations to make. It should be self-evident that different talents, interests, and paths need to be encouraged in children. In the big concert of all well-intentioned souls on this planet, each soul should learn to play his or her own instrument fluently. Only then will the music sound harmonious to everyone.

When children have very different Signatures among their siblings, it is important to encourage individuality, since many situations can arise in which one child confuses his or her talents for inadequacies. You should never measure the failure of one child against the success of the other. Nor should you give a child the impression that he or she is flawed or of lesser value, especially when report card results vary widely. One could be an early starter and the other a late bloomer. One could constantly strive to win while the other is indifferent, measuring his or her own success with a different ruler. One may be a quick learner, while the other retains things longer. The list goes on.

With the Code, parents ideally learn to be the wise conductors of a band that takes pleasure in the diversity of its members. Would a guitar player tell a drummer, "My guitar playing is way better than your drum playing?" No. The guitar and drums are two completely different instruments. But when they are played together in an orchestrated fashion, the sum is greater than its parts. Likewise, you cannot compare one Signature against the other. The point is for the two Signatures to play their best and in close collaboration in order to make a beautiful and harmonious sound for the good of us all. The Code is a wonderful instrument in the hands of a sage conductor. It is best to allow togetherness to mature while encouraging your children to appreciate their differences.

Timing is one of the most important skills of a conductor *and* a parent. For small children, the application of their Signature colors should prevail. With older children, a wise selection of reading material related to their Numbers is important for grabbing their interest and attention. It is also vital to have age-appropriate conversations with children who frequently point out the reason for seemingly unfair conduct on the parent's part—in other words, children are treated on an individual basis according to age, ability, and interests. When the age difference between children is large, it does not really matter. But problems can arise when there is an age difference of only one or two years. As just one of many examples, it helped us to instruct our younger child to do the same homework as her older sibling if she wanted to stay up just as late, which helped her understand age-appropriate responsibilities better and learn what is fair.

When raising children, consider the existing Cardinal Points as well as the voids; developing the missing Stations of a Signature is relatively easy to do (see part 2 for suggestions). Just learn more about what is missing. Is it the vibrancy of the South, the adaptability of the East, the balance of the Center, the healthy egotism and willpower of the West, or the plethora of ideas of the North? Using the knowledge of the Code, you can give your children a promising start in life. It is never too early to start conquering the missing Stations that complete the overall picture.

◆ ◆ A Story from Johanna ◆ ◆

After the birth of my first son, I used the time at home to tutor neighborhood children—mostly children with learning difficulties who spoke no German. I well remember an eleven-year-old boy who, during one of our first meetings, paced up and down like a little tiger in front of my living room window, mumbling, "When I'm eighteen, I am going to kill them all." I stood there helplessly for a few seconds, and then I knew that something had to be done, and soon. The father had been an academic in his native country and put tremendous pressure on his oldest son to become a success. But he did so without taking into account the boy's talents, his Signature, and his frame of mind. The child barely spoke German and received no encouragement whatsoever in school. At home, he was fighting a losing battle, and he was about to repeat the second grade. Of course, in their way, teachers were "right" in letting him fail; the father was "right"; and the son was also "right" in his hatred. So now what?

Normally, I prefer using the individual biorhythm when working with a child (see our book *Moon Time*, page 227). Improvement is usually quick with children, and from then on, they stop feeling overtaxed and start succeeding in school, often for the first time. With this child, it was not possible to do this. His exact day of birth was unknown, so neither biorhythms nor the Code would fully work. However, I did know the year of his birth—19**7****4**—which helped a lot. This was a child who had spirit and a desire for success, but patience was not his strongest point. I could also see that underneath all that hatred was a great ability to love. In tune with the requirements of developing the talents of the West and the South, we practiced hands-on learning, which was outdoors as much as possible and used a variety of practical examples. For math, I literally worked with apple halves! With the help of the Code, I was able to prevent the resignation in this child from turning into rage.

We have all come across such aggressions. Some children who love freedom more than being sheltered become aggressive against overly protective parents. Do not automatically pity latchkey children, because some of them thrive in the absence of controlling parents. On the other hand, children who want to be intensely cared for may develop aggressions against their negligent parents, joining any kind of group that promises togetherness and harmony. Numerous far-right and far-left groups, as well as religious sects, exist only because they exploit the most beautiful human qualities: the innate longing for togetherness and the desire to be in good hands. The real differences between these seducers dwell only in the heads of people who profit from such differentiations. Political labels merely serve to obscure the true circumstances.

The solution is never to complain or justify endlessly; the solution is always inner contentment. Learn not to hold others responsible for your situation, and take charge of your destiny. With the help of the Code, you can do just that.

Now why is it so important to me to devote a few lines to these interrelations? Because it is true that war and terror are nothing more than an uprising against injustice, whether it is on a small or large scale, in the fate of a single person or the fate of an entire nation. Shortly after an injustice has been committed, no one is interested in the reasons why this individual or group of people started to fight back. In their blind fixation on symptoms, the media show only the spectacular outcomes of uprisings and of acts of terror. Thus, they frequently depict a situation incorrectly and bring irrelevancies to the forefront. If they continue to report only about the aftermath, the symptoms, and the riotous behavior, it is understandable that everyone is calling out to wage war against terror. But this battle will never be successful. Instead, it will result in more suffering and misery for generations to come.

Politicians who pretend to want to "fight evil" instead of making a serious effort to discover the roots of injustice in day-to-day life are dangerous. Their focus is on votes and self-aggrandizement, and they ruin far more in the world than the denounced bad guys. We face a greater danger when we deliberately keep people in the dark so that they vote a certain way. Have we not elected enough windbags into office? When we fail to see the connections between what we reap and what we sow, we will continue to blame others and will never feel free. Freedom and dignity have to do with having a heart and not with national boundaries or material goods. The Code can provide a step toward freedom—namely, to help you live the life that was meant to be yours from the very beginning.

All of us need to change our mental routines to put an end to injustice and exploitation. Start with yourself, and you will see what a giant step it is. The Numbers on the Birthday Wheel tell you exactly where to begin and which friends—those who offer the beneficial qualities of their Signatures—can be of help. In this way, children and adults alike replace aggression with inner contentment.

"He who has the gold makes the rules." There is hardly a proverb that is truer or more depressing. But we don't have to join in. That is the secret weapon—the remedy that all of us can use if only we choose to. If we live for the good in us, the world will also change for the good. We are absolutely certain that this is so. Share our certainty, and join us in taking action!

The Numbers of the Century and the Millennium

Although the Numbers of the century and the millennium in which we live play a secondary role in how to use a Signature, we had promised you that we would talk a bit about their meaning. These two Numbers are more important for the effect that they have on mankind than for the impact they have on individuals.

Here is some food for thought: Have you noticed that World War I and World War II began in the years of the dispassionate West (191❹ and 193❾) and ended with the Numbers of the compassionate East and the balancing Center (191❽ and 194❺)? The bundled energy of the ❶ and ❾ in their negative expressions surely contributed to the twentieth century having such a warrior image. The "dark sides" of the ❶ and ❾ brought aggression, the desire to stubbornly assert oneself right down to the bitter end, the pollution of the environment and mind, egotism, emotional dependence, and physical addiction. Ricarda Winterswyl commented on this in an article published in *Süddeutsche Zeitung*, a German newspaper, on April 20, ❶❾❾❶:

Citizens are becoming increasingly dependent on services that they cannot influence and on experts who advise them and tell them how to live. Man's normal, inborn abilities suffocate under the onslaught of regulations and instructions. As a result, man remains dependent like a child. He is both allowed to and expected to remain that way. He no longer believes in himself, the future, or in the self-regulating power of life.

(Translated by Thomas Poppe)

What does the twenty-first century have in store for us? Above all, hope! The ❷ and ⓪ stand for warmhearted balance and harmony, indicating renewal and a new beginning. It means taking a step back to the Center. Starting around 2030, the children born in 2000 will start repairing what we destroyed. The self-centered twentieth century (❶ and ❾) will give way to the ❷ and ⓪, which have the power to move and combine disparate energies. These two Numbers ensure that children born now will start to iron out the mistakes of their parents and grandparents. The laziness and mental inertia of the consumer society will be replaced with something better. And globalization will change from being a symbol for exploitation and coldness to a symbol for the celebration of harmonious cooperation and multiracial world cultures.

A millennium has a slow but steady influence as it shapes all of mankind. It will take a while before the effect of the ❷ and ⓪ is felt. However, the groundwork is in place for the return of reason. Political booby traps and empty promises will be more easily recognized; personal responsibility will have more value; the consumer's buying frenzy will abate; and the emphasis on true value and quality will grow. As we said, it will take a while, and those of us who are the border crossers between the two centuries can start immediately to give it our best effort. Without saying a word, simply turn your back on those naysayers who claim that a single person cannot achieve or change anything; even when acting alone, every single person can change something. An individual who follows a good path can have tremendous influence—look at Gandhi. Perhaps there will soon be many more remarkable individuals like him!

The Code and Geography

In addition to these brief instructions concerning the Signatures with respect to everyday life, we would like to expand a little on a topic that we brought up at the beginning of the book: the Geographic Signature. Each artificial separation of homogenous nations or dissolution of national boundaries brings with it political and human upheaval, as well as profound changes in the living organism that is a country. The residents of a municipality, town, or country form their own organic identities to a much greater degree than we tend to realize. They develop independent characters. Many a traveler has encountered this but without fully understanding the true reason for it.

This is the main reason why people who willingly change from their own culture to a new one (for whatever reason) quickly adjust and feel at home once they have assimilated to the customs, eating habits, and other aspects of their new home and culture. Those who stubbornly cling to the lifestyle of their former homeland end up feeling homeless and uprooted.

The former eastern corner of West Germany, for example, had to come to grips with being located in the Center of Germany after the fall of the Berlin Wall. It was now assigned the Numbers ❶ and ❺ and the color yellow. After World War I, instead of being located in the South of Austria, South Tyrol became a province of Northern Italy with the stroke of a pen, and then took over the tasks of the ❻ and ❶. To this day, many of South Tyrol's citizens do not consider themselves to be Italians. We hope that this book will inspire you to discover what your own geographic interrelations mean for you personally in your own adventure through life. It is a rewarding, worthwhile task to watch the ramifications of such dynamic movement.

Let's consider a few more examples to help you address this topic on your own.

Imagine a family named Awaywego moves from one part of the United States to another—let's say from Portland, Oregon, to Miami, Florida. How the family and its individual members adjust to their new environment depends on numerous factors—weather, time zone, cuisine, and so on. It is also important to consider the geographical aspects of the Birthday Wheel and how the directions of the compass relate to existing Cardinal Points in one's Signature. Many people underestimate how a feeling of belonging evolves, what the determining factors are, and why its positive development takes a long time or never occurs.

One of the reasons lies in the individual locations of people's dwellings. It is sometimes more problematic to move from the North of town to the South of town than to move from the North of one continent (Sweden, for example) to the North of another continent (say, Canada). The feeling that drove the Awaywego family to Miami, or people from Canada to Mexico, or retirees from New York to California, has its roots in such energy interplays.

Moving can be a happy and successful step for a family, but sometimes it is a leap from the frying pan into the fire. We may unconsciously want to escape the energy of the North (❻/❶) by moving South (❼/❷). However, if we move to the northern part of a southern city, we could encounter the same energy that we were trying to avoid. If the Awaywegos move from Portland, Oregon, to the northern part of Miami, they may discover that, after months and years of living there, the old wanderlust returns. On the other hand, provided they pay close attention to the energies of the Geographic Signature of Miami, their vital need to belong someplace will definitely be satisfied.

The ramifications of these energies in the day-to-day life of individuals are honed with each geographic dimension—from continent to country, from region to town, from one individual's dwelling to another. It could be that you feel very comfortable living in the eastern part of a town, but your bedroom or home office is located in the West of your house. You may love your town but are simply not comfortable at home.

In the same way, if your date of birth has a lot of East (❽/❸), then it might not be good for you to live on the East side of town for a long period of time. The eastern part of a country can also get on your nerves. If you cannot move, then you should at least choose a bedroom or a home office that is not located on the East side of your home. The same principle can be applied to all other Numbers in a date of birth.

Going deeper into the microcosm, we find that even if a room faces the right way, the direction we face in that room also has an influence. For example, when your date of birth has an extreme Center of Gravity in the North, you might find that you sleep restlessly in the North of your bedroom. These are just some ways that playing with geographic locations can provide additional insight into your Numbers and help you find the happiness you've been looking for. Sometimes it is enough to move into a home across the street to quell a lifelong wanderlust, or to move your bed to the other side of the room to get a peaceful night of sleep.

It is entirely possible for members of the Awaywego family to find their happiness in the place of their choosing, and we wish this for them and for anyone who dares to take that step. Remember, however, that sometimes moving your bed is all it takes to find and keep this happiness.

The Power of the Actual Date

A long time ago, it was common to use the energy of the Numbers and the Signature Stations in many areas of life and work. We would like to introduce you to a few of these situations, as we encourage you to gather your own experiences with this tool. And while our recommendations might not sound current, they do offer an interesting way to see the big picture when using the Code and the individual rules of conduct.

You say your Signature has a strong East (❽/❸)? In that case, it is important to be careful with wood (such as carving, carpentry, siding, roofing, and so on) on days with an ❽ or ❸ in the actual date. For example, if a farmer decides to work with wood anyway, he should make sure that someone who has a ❾ or ❹ accompanies him in his task. He should also wear protective gear, like a helmet, safety boots, gloves, and so on, since the risk of getting hurt is greater on these days. And any storms occurring on days with an ❽ or ❸ are apt to cause more extensive damage than on other days.

What if the day's date has a ❼ or ❷? On those days, people with a Signature that has the Center of Gravity in the South should not exert themselves. For example, they should not plan deliveries or long car trips on ❼ or ❷ days. Dangerous trips into the mountains (and similar adventures) should also be avoided, and working a long time in the sun is also more dangerous on these days. In the past, people whose Signature had a heavily populated South were sent into the shade to avoid heat strokes and fevers, and children got even more protection from the sun. If the moon happens to be in Leo, the effect intensifies because Leo is the fieriest, "driest" of all Zodiac signs. Firemen should also use extra caution on Leo days, as accidents from fires will be more devastating. The fire will burn stronger and will spread more quickly; campfires must also be watched closely. Most forest fires occur in July (❼) and not in August, and the damage in July tends to be greater.

On days with a ❾ or ❹ in the actual date, a person of the West should not make dangerous repairs on machinery. Instead, it should be left to a person with a ❻ or ❶ in his or her birthdate. In the distant past, this knowledge helped prevent serious industrial accidents. For example, new machinery was used for the first time only on days that did not have a ❾ or ❹ in the actual date. On all other days, bearers of the West Signature were very welcome, even for manual tasks or repairs.

On days of the North (days in which the actual date contains a ❻ or ❶), a person of the North should relinquish the ship's helm to another person when on a major sea voyage. You should also not sail or dive on those days, and spelunkers must be very careful to avoid all risks. In the global climate, the ❻ and ❶ represent "cold" and "damp." This is one reason why we tend to have floods on certain days in January and June.

What if the actual date contains mostly Numbers of the Center (⓿ and ❺)? In that case, you should merely take good care of your money or someone else's instead of trying to increase monetary wealth—especially if you, too, have a ⓿ of ❺ in your date of birth. Every extra influence of the Center makes you more arrogant and miserly on those days, and in an extreme case, can make you ill.

◆   ◆   ◆   ◆   ◆

We were happy to provide you with the Signature sketches of part 3 and the color palettes of part 2. Now it is up to you to provide the fine brush needed to work out the pictures, their dynamics, their bursts of color, and their rich details. We hope this chapter provided you with ideas for doing just that.

14

How to Get Well and Stay Well Using the Code

One of the oldest and noblest of all arts is healing and keeping people healthy. The healers, shamans, and medicine men of our ancestors were held in the highest esteem, and those who go through life with open eyes today know that this reverence is still alive—and for the most part, rightfully so. Simultaneously, however, a grave change has taken place under the starched white surfaces of modern physicians' coats as a result of the explosive arrival of a certain form of knowledge acquisition—one that holds the tools of healing in higher regard than the permanent success of their application.

For decades, the pharmaceutical industry has wanted you to believe that healthcare is its business and no one else's, attempting to take a place of influence similar to that of the Church in earlier years. It wants to monopolize healing in order to have power and to create dependence.

True healing (done with the help of conscious awareness and by the removal of illnesses' root causes) has taken a step back or even gone underground—to the benefit of symptom-driven medicine. There is little to challenge modern providers who are satisfied when the headache is gone and the tonsils are out. Their focus is on medications, machines, X-rays, surgeries, and vaccinations.

Gradually, a new generation of true healers and friends of humankind is returning to the scene, thanks in part to the ❷ and ⓪ of the new Millennium. The road to vitality and success is coming to meet you, dear reader! Even though you did not grow up with the experiences and the information found in this book, you have the right and the opportunity to benefit from them.

Please note that we do not want to give you the idea that the Birthday Wheel is a panacea; if the body decides to become healthy, small details can tip the scales. However, if it does not trust its captain, namely, your spirit, it will go into a downward spiral. With this book, we have tried to provide many of the powerful details that were used in our day-to-day life with the Birthday Wheel. To go into greater detail and eventualities would fill an additional book, so we have limited ourselves to some related ideas and information we consider helpful in this last part of the book. We guarantee that its remedies will work—and without any negative side effects!

◆ ◆ A Story from Johanna ◆ ◆

I was fifteen years old when I decided to leave our farm to go to Munich to learn, learn, learn whatever the big world had to offer.

Since such a step was not common in our village, I had special difficulties to face. The first one was the image of women at that time. People thought that a girl did not need to learn anything because she was only meant to serve—whomever or whatever. Second, my parents made it clear that I could not simply return home if I failed, and that did not make my decision any easier.

However, I was not prepared for the biggest problem I would encounter. At fifteen, I was strong as a horse and knew what I had to do in order to stay healthy. By the time I was eighteen and had lived in the city for three years, I had chronic gastritis and my vision had deteriorated. Among other things, I needed glasses, and for the first time in my life, I had to see a physician. When I did, I was appalled by how little a city doctor knew about the true connections between things.

I had reached a dead end because I no longer ate healthy, organic food and no longer paid attention to the phases of the moon. I became both physically and mentally weak, but I wanted to belong at any price. Being "old-fashioned" just did not fit the bill.

Years would pass before I once again lived by nature's rhythms, and at first, I only did so in secret. After much suffering, I found my way back to the right path—but not without ridicule from those who are unfamiliar with this type of knowledge. I have never taken the much-traveled road, so it did not bother me greatly. Today, I'm back on the road of personal responsibility, and that road is not a major highway. Many who have not found their way yet can discover it more easily by using the Code. Above all, they can gain the strength to stay on their chosen path.

Every person has his or her individual way of regenerating. One person needs the mountains to regain strength and joy in life, while another would almost perish at those heights. One person must have water, lakes, and the ocean but cannot stand the heat. Another catches a cold at the mere thought of cool waters and would rather relax on a warm beach. Some people need dry heat in order to recharge their inner batteries. It also happens that some people need the hustle and bustle of a big city in order to feel alive—there is a reason why city living is so expensive. The city gives many people the feeling that all is right with the world. People take the subway to work; cabs are blowing their horns; stores are open. The city never sleeps, so city people feel alive with vitality.

Everyone lives their Numbers, their Signature, and their unique life as it relates to the Code—one of the most beneficial tools for getting well and staying well, even in this day and age. It is sad that today's medicine and science only affirms that something is good and right if that method heals anyone at any time. Unfortunately, this merely suppresses symptoms, if that. Modern logic combined with a strict adherence to statistics can destroy more than it helps build. If you want to lead a full life, you need to look beyond today's conventional wisdom to that of the past.

The decisive factors for a healthy immune system are the phases of regeneration, but it is important that regeneration actually takes place. The way that this occurs differs from person to person and cannot be limited to one universal method. One person regains her strength by retreating and spending time alone, while another person revives by being around his family. Yet another needs work, motorcycle races, or chess to regenerate. Your date of birth and your Signature will show you the fastest and most successful way to regenerate and stay well.

To give a few examples, people who have a lot of North (❻/❶) in their Signature often love water for regenerating and strengthening their immune system, but it does not necessarily have to be the ocean. A mountain stream or a lake is usually sufficient, and vacations are an efficient (and fun) way to find this balance and strength for the entire year.

People whose Center of Gravity is located in the South (❼/❷) sometimes prefer cooler regions, especially those with an excess of Numbers in the South (more than ten units). The vibrant people of the South are frequently passionate mountain climbers as well. On a side note, bearers should avoid vacationing in a hot climate during July since the ❼ adds to the heat. In August (❽), 85°F does not have the same effect as 85°F the month before. Paying attention to such details prevents unnecessary heat-related problems.

Someone who loves the ocean does not necessarily have to love heat. Maybe you can better understand now why some people prefer a cooler ocean beach or the cascading waters of a mountain stream, while others love the hot wind on Southern waters. Families often have heated discussions about the right destination. It would only be fair to take turns from year to year, visiting various climates.

You run the risk of weakening your immune system when you regularly take vacations in countries that are not suited for you, especially if you do this merely to please your partner. It is also important to know that when two people have a Number in common in their date of birth, it creates a certain harmony. However, the shared South (❼/❷) in their dates of birth does not automatically mean that they should both vacation in northern regions. Perhaps it is enough to vacation at the seashore once a year to allow the South to recoup its energies. You could also spend an entire weekend in the garden. For a Signature with a strong Center (0 / 5), this is often more than adequate to recharge all the batteries. Draw your own conclusions; they can be easily transferred to other Signatures. Nothing in the realm of the Code is ever only good or only bad.

Our immune system does best when we have the feeling that we are doing something useful. This could be staying strong and healthy, looking forward to an event, saving for something, burning with desire, or living in an environment where we feel understood! The worst poison for our immune system is not being understood. Some people get to be one hundred years old by happily anticipating one thing after another—advancing from daily goal to daily goal, weekly goal to weekly goal; making resolutions year after year; attaining life goal after life goal. Great healers often report how the life of terminally ill patients was prolonged and improved when they had new ambitions—getting a belated degree, seeing a once-in-a-lifetime concert of one's favorite band, writing a mystery novel, getting a prize for having the most beautiful roses in the neighborhood.

You weaken your immune system—this glowing globe of light and colors around each of us—when you do not live your Numbers or fill your Signature with life. Even when you live your Numbers, things might not always go smoothly for you, but you will be far healthier and more fulfilled than you would have ever been by blindly following ingrained habits. What progress this would be to discover that when you are not feeling well, are depressed, or have lost your passion, you are merely not living your Number treasure—it helps a lot! But we have to walk on our own two feet to get the winnings.

Healing with the Code

The following examples will help you embark on a journey of discovery through the broad spectrum of possibilities offered by the Code. Healers (and those with an interest in healing) would be especially happy to get this information, for it will explain many strange events in day-to-day life.

Let's assume that you or someone you know is ill. The first step is to look at the personal Signature involved. Where is the Center of Gravity? Where are the Numbers most heavily concentrated? Which Stations are missing?

Healing with the South

Let's assume that the person in question was born on May 25, 1972. You see immediately that the element of heat is heavily weighted with one ❼ and two ❷s in the South. Based upon that, it is highly likely that a fever will be the main defense mechanism of this immune system. A fever's function is to keep pathogens at bay and eventually kill them. When this person has a temperature of 101°F, it is advisable to let the fever spike instead of reaching for fever-reducing medications. People of the South react to illness by quickly developing a fever and respond positively to cool water, cold compresses, and other cooling methods. However, we need to be aware that cold compresses are not always called for. There are times when different medical treatments are definitely the better solution.

One of the special characteristics of the people of the South is that as long as they get enough exercise, they have great resistance to illness. However, they need true rest in order to make a quick recovery. If a person of the South is physically still but distracts himself by watching TV or by reading, it will delay the healing process. Standing still does not mean that people of the South are resting—not in daily life and not on vacation. They need to truly rest their mind and body.

Let us quickly take another step and combine these ways of healing with the actual date on which the illness occurs; the importance and meaning of doing this should not be underestimated. For example, let's take a patient with a heavy South (lots of ❼s or ❷s) who has frequent fevers, often without any discernible cause. Here is a hint to train your powers of observation: this person gets a fever more frequently on days that contain a lot of ❼s or ❷s. Strange parallels, aren't they?

If you have a child who has a lot of South in his or her Signature, 2007 was not an easy year. The same held true for all people whose immune systems responded to pathogens with fever. Generally, such a child will be more prone to have a fever on days that have a lot of ❼s or ❷s rather than at other times. This tendency can stabilize when those around this child are mindful of it. Gradually, it will no longer matter which day it is.

Healing with the North

Let's assume that a person's North (❻/❶), Center (0 / 5), and South (❼/❷) have Numbers, but only one ❷ is present. However, there are many Units in the North (for example, two ❻s). In that circumstance, the onset of a fever as a defense mechanism is not an initial response, but this person of the North will feel sick as dog once the fever starts. Apply cold compresses sooner rather than later.

A person of the North finds it difficult to tolerate idleness of any kind—that includes bed rest. The people of the North risk harm by standing still and motionless, but as a necessary part of their therapy, they should lie down or only move around moderately.

A person whose Signature has a heavy North feels best when they drink lots of liquids. This is in complete harmony with water, the element of the North, and people of the North can be healed with it. When there is too much energy in the North, the opposite South should be asked to help—a lot of warmth (bed, sauna, and so on). The drink of choice would be lots of tea, and an herbal bath would also serve well. These remedies may differ from person to person, however.

Some people need to find a way to deal with fluid retention. For this, you should select a day with a numerical date that contains plenty of energy from the South (❼/❷). On that day, nothing should be consumed but diuretic tea. If you were to do this on a day with a lot of North (❻/❶), it would not be nearly as successful (perhaps not successful at all).

As you have seen so often before, success depends on your intentions. Detoxifying and diuretic treatments for example (as shown in our other books) will be far more effective when done during a waning moon. Wisely combining all influences will result in faster healing. It takes skillful handling.

Here, as everywhere in life, the correct amount of a remedy is vital. As we mentioned before, it is important to know that a person with a strong

South can deal well with a fever and may even need one to get well. If the fever is reduced too soon, the person will frequently react with another. In other words, in order to heal, this person has to truly utilize and savor the fever. For the typical person of the North, the opposite holds true. That person is more receptive to tea and to healing with water. However, constantly drinking tea is not indicated for everyone in every situation. A hot bath and hot tea followed by a warm bed can do wonders. But a fever-ish person of the North needs cooling down in order to get well. Of course, we are not suggesting that you let this person lie near an open window! We are, however, recommending cooling with cold (never ice-cold) compresses, frequent washing of the face, leg ice packs, and so on. Herbal baths can also be effective here. As usual, all things should be done in moderation.

Healing with the East

In former times, it was customary to tailor treatments to the need of the individual. Ingredients and supplies for various treatment methods were kept on hand as a matter of course. The fermenting of herbs was as natural as steeping medicinal herbs in alcohol or preparing ointments from pork lard and herbs.

People with an East (❽/❸) Center of Gravity benefit most from fermented herbs. (During fermentation, ingredients undergo a chemical conversion with the help of enzymes or bacteria.) For example, as a preventive or treatment for cough, ribwort was put in a jar and covered with sugar. The jar was then buried in the ground until the fermentation process was complete. This supply would last the entire winter. In case you would like to try this recipe, you should use the resulting syrup the way you would use honey: either take it straight on a teaspoon, or you can dissolve it in tea or other drinks. The taste is not to everyone's liking, so children often need much praise and encouragement for their brave behavior when taking the ribwort and doing what is good for them. But it is well worth the effort, as this remedy is far superior to most products found in a pharmacy.

Children with a more heavily weighted Center in their Signature (**0** / **5**) used to have salve rubbed on their chests for the same symptoms. When the actual date displayed a lot of energy of the East, the treatment method was different from when it was done on West (**9**/**4**) or South (**7**/**2**) days.

Children and adults whose Center of Gravity is located in the East require peace and quiet in order to get back on their feet. At the same time, they need plenty of fresh air since their lungs and their respiratory systems are often vulnerable. The illnesses of the people of the East are often carried by the wind.

Healing with the West

For people with the West in their Signature (**9**/**4**), a small glass of wine is good medicine. Herbal elixirs with an alcoholic base also do wonders for them. As always, this is not appropriate for every case; for example, people whose date of birth contains too much of the North's (**6**/**1**) energy rarely tolerate alcoholic remedies well. On occasion, they may even breed an alcoholic addiction. You should be especially concerned about children here. In certain instances, the absence of the energy of the North leads to the same potential problems with alcohol. Someone who helps himself to a hearty dinner every day and follows it up with a strong herbal digestive surely misses the true purpose of this remedy.

Here is another secret of the West: too much lying around is never the most effective way to be fit. There are always exceptions, but in general, a lack of exercise will harm a person of the West. Stomach, intestines, and muscles need an active body, and this is often the weak spot for a person of the West. A person's meridians unite and harmonize through movement, which is even more pronounced in this Station. If you keep moving, you will rarely become ill. And if you do become ill, it will most likely be an accident that lays you up. You won't remain horizontal for too long, though; the people of the West bounce back quickly and are back on their feet soon after an operation. Although you should not overdo this good quality, when your instincts tell you to get up, follow them. Just use caution.

Healing with the Center

The Numbers and the methods of the Center (**0** / **5**) stand in very close relationship to the centers of our bodies and, therefore, have an impact on all the organs that are affected in 80 percent of all illnesses. In order for the body to stay healthy, all the detoxifying organs, all the glands, the heart, and the lungs must function. You should not miss taking measures to strengthen these organs on days with a **0** or **5** in the actual date—or at least avoid stress and strain on those days.

The people of the Center would do well to pay attention to healthy nutrition in order to pamper their inner organs. Many aches and illnesses could be avoided if the people of the Center recognized these important connections early on. Their bodies are the fastest to recover as long as they eat organic food and avoid animal protein. Fast food puts a strain on everyone's body, but the effect on people of the Center is even greater. For them, vegetables marinated in organic oil and fresh fruit are not only a culinary delight but they speed the recovery process. Unfortunately, most plant oils sold in supermarkets have been chemically processed and are more harmful than helpful. If you use only cold-pressed organic oils, you will soon find that oil can be medicinal. If you are familiar with our books on nutrition, you will appreciate the fact that even butter can heal (see our website www.paungger-poppe.com).

People of the Center require a slow, comfortable rest during the healing and recovery period. (Just the opposite of people of the West.) If a person of the Center knows the self and body well, he or she will be incomprehensible to the hectic and fiery characters among us (the South [**7**/**2**] in particular). The Center heals and regenerates when it is able to move slowly and peacefully—at a snail's pace. On the surface it seems that nothing can ruffle its feathers. Maybe our forebears had the gentle people of the Center in mind when they honored their achievements in the proverb "A horse is faster than the wind, but the faithful camel trudges through the desert, day and night."

Too little sleep does the greatest damage to the liver and the gall-bladder, since both organs regenerate between 1 AM and 3 AM. Perhaps this is the reason for your liver problems? Are you getting too little rest because your toddler interrupts your sleep? Do you have a person in the family in need of constant care? Are too many worries keeping you awake?

Meditation is an important element in the healing process for the person of the Center; too much worry literally makes him or her sick. For this reason, you should meditate and pray on a date that holds a lot of Center (0 / 5) energy. We all have our own access to a Higher Power, but you are the one who has to take the initiative to open the door.

By all means, try one or more of the suggestions in this chapter, especially if you are in a healing profession. These secrets are surprisingly timeless and valid. In the past, people used—and were thankful for—everything nature had to offer. We need to return to that approach. If we do, then perhaps the pharmaceutical industry will make people-friendly remedies produced in harmony with nature.

Once Upon a Time: Wound Healing in Accordance with the Code

The information we are about to share with you is rarely used in this day and age, though, in our experience, it has not lost any of its value. The basic principles of staying healthy and of healing are also accessible in the methodology of the Code. The next discussion deals specifically with cleverly devised procedures used in earlier times for dealing with poorly healing wounds.

These wounds, especially open leg wounds and other similar problems, are almost always an external sign of blood poisoning. The customary methods of treatment in such cases were special poultices, often with frequently changed herbal recipes, and any such remedy was formulated in accordance with a specific date. Close attention was paid to the following:

The Phase of the Moon

All treatments took place during a waning moon to maximize the long-term effect. During a waning moon, the body detoxifies more quickly and wounds heal better. During a waxing moon, the healing process slows down, increasing the likelihood of infection. Extra precautions were also taken; meticulous cleanliness, for one, was of utmost importance.

The Moon in the Zodiac

The Zodiac signs in the moon calendar can intensify or weaken the effect of therapy. Each of the twelve zodiacal influences rules a certain part of the body—from Aries to Pisces, from head to toe. The advice here is to avoid the Zodiac signs that govern the part of the body that is being treated. For example, an open wound on the lower leg should not be treated during Aquarius. Details about prevention and healing in harmony with the rhythms of the moon and of nature can be found in our book *Moon Time*.

Selecting Medicinal Herbs

It is important that the type and quantity of a medicinal herb and the time of application are in balance. First you need to determine if the plant should have a detoxifying, astringent, anti-inflammatory, anticonvulsant, or other effect. For example, the very common plant ribwort plantain (*Plantago lanceolata*) is not only anti-inflammatory but, when put on an open wound, can treat blood poisoning. The bandage used should be changed twice during a waning moon and once during a waxing moon. (The waning moon has a detoxifying effect; during a waxing moon, it is best to leave the wound alone.)

Changing your Eating Habits

Without a change in eating habits, treatment of poorly healing wounds often fails, since these wounds are usually symptoms of blood poisoning. Today, as in the past, incorrect eating habits are related to the cause. In the past, no milk products or animal protein in any form was allowed during healing. Of course, the treatment also depended on the nutritional type of the person—whether he or she was type Alpha or Omega, for example. Compensating for mineral or vitamin deficiencies by taking these elements in their pure forms is virtually useless; the body is inefficient when it comes to absorbing food, mineral, and vitamin supplements. We can get the vital nutrients our body needs only from organic vegetables and fruit. (Homeopathic Schuessler cell salts could also be helpful here.)

Disposing of Used Bandages in Harmony with a Specific Date
This is where it gets tricky, as the precise method of disposing of the bandages also has an impact on whether or not the wound heals successfully. The disposal should be timed with the personal Signature of the patient and the date of the treatment, which is explained in the text that follows.

◆ **Treatment on Days with a ❻ or ❶**
The days with the North (❻ or ❶) are generally well suited for water treatment. In the aftermath of a burn wound, the old bandages should be disposed of outdoors in a watery environment. (In the past, the bandages were buried under the drain pipe.) However, it is sufficient to bury them anywhere in the ground as long as the area is watered. It is crucial that the bandages decompose in a moist environment.

◆ **Treatment on Days with an ❽ or a ❸**
In the case of gangrene and on treatment days with the East (days with an ❽ or a ❸ in the date), bandages are disposed of in an acidic environment. This disposes of the illness regardless of what kind of disposing acid is used. (Children should be kept away from this work so that they do not get hurt.) Long ago, the bandages were drenched with vinegar and buried far away. Another past method

involved placing the bandage on an anthill to be eaten. Today, we would not recommend this method with these small valuable creatures, as it seems more like animal cruelty to us.

- **Treatment on Days with a ❼ or ❷**

  When dealing with a festering wound on days with a ❼ or ❷ in the date, ideally, the bandages are burned. If there is ample sun, extreme exposure in the sunlight produces excellent results. But in any case, the bandage has to dry and cannot come into contact with water.

- **Treatment on Days with a ❾ or ❹**

  On these days, the illness can be chased away by burning incense. Smoke is thought to help fight germs, and the healing process usually starts very quickly. Great care has to be taken that every room is vented to the outside, and keeping the outside doors and windows open does the job. If burning incense was not possible in the past, the bandages went to decompose on the dunghill.

- **Treatment on Days with a ⓪ or ⑤**

  The Numbers and the methods of the Center call for burying everything in accordance with this Station's earthy energy.

As long as these five bandage disposal rules were observed, successful healing was the norm more than the exception. This was the case with stubborn, chronic conditions and ailments among the elderly as well.

At this point, you probably wonder if these strange methods for the disposal of bandages really make sense. What mechanism is at work here?

Whether or not an injury heals depends upon powers and elements that can elude the scientifically trained eye. Your new knowledge from this book adds important components to your personal tool chest when it comes to the challenges of life, not just when it relates to healing. Healing is more than a physio-chemical process; heart and mind also play roles here.

Until recently, the World Health Organization officially defined health as the "absence of illness," but that's only part of it. First, and above all, health means the strength and ability that every person requires to become what their Higher Power envisioned for them. Second, health means having the ability to reject and overcome what is keeping us from becoming that envisioned person. Third, it describes a condition of life that comes from harmonious, dynamic synergy among body, mind, soul, and the world.

Our ancestors knew these interrelations and the necessities that arose from them. Healers, shamans, and medicine men knew that people were more than physical machines; they knew that the body, mind, and soul formed a whole. They also knew that the whole was irrevocably inter-linked with our surroundings—other people, nature, and even the stars. People become ill when they lose the momentum to balance the many elements in life—between tension and relaxation, a healthy egotism and surrender, and the ups and downs of fate. Healing masters of the past knew how to regain this balance when it was lost and how important it was that a human was a being composed of energies.

◆　◆　◆　◆　◆

The fact that everything in nature is energy was known long before Albert Einstein articulated it. Ancient cultures also knew that everything is sound, oscillation, and rhythm, and that our body consists of color and light. The apparently solid parts are merely a form of intensive illusion—a lucid dream. Physicists discovered some time ago that each individual cell gives off light, and that it is possible to make this light visible. Further, it changes when the condition of the cell changes.

The long-term scientific world view is both sad and meaningless, as it has done little to incorporate Einstein's realization into the education of health professionals. Medical schools are extremely reluctant to accept that the body houses feelings, thoughts, and instincts that all play a big role where illness is concerned. It is even rarer to hear medical professionals acknowledges that thoughts and feelings also heal, let alone see them engage in the ongoing development of such methods.

Yet we have all experienced this firsthand. How do we feel when we are in love? We are ready to take on anything! Do you know anyone who became ill in the midst of falling in love?

How do we feel when we are depressed, suffer from stress, or are desperate? What had cooled in our soul the last time we caught a cold? We know all the connections and do not need textbooks to verify them. They tell us only one thing: health is a matter of many various energies and connections.

"Strange" things happen in nature. They have all been proven scientifically and can be easily duplicated, but they cannot all be explained with modern methods.

- When pests attack trees at the edge of a forest, the affected trees produce certain chemicals in self-defense. Not only that, but simultaneously, the trees at the other end of the forest react the same way, even though the arrival of the pest is still a few weeks away.
- When kittens are taken too early from the mother cat, they barely learn to catch mice, if at all. They remain amateur hunters for a long time. If you put these incapable kittens into a cage at night to sleep in the same room with caged cats who are experienced hunters (so that the experienced cats cannot demonstrate their hunting skills), the young cats learn within a few days how to catch mice without ever having seen it.
- Before a plant expert took a long trip to Europe, he wired the large leaves of his favorite houseplant (a monstera) to numerous instruments to measure all sorts of electrical currents in the plant. While in Europe, he kept a diary in which he made note of high stress situations—when he was stuck in traffic, shortly before a big speech, a split second of fear, and so on. When he returned home after six weeks, he discovered that the measuring devices on his monstera had spiked during those moments when he was under great stress in Europe.

♦ A nursing mother is visiting a neighbor miles away, and her baby is peacefully sleeping at home. Suddenly, in the middle of the conversation, the mother starts lactating, and at the same time, the baby wakes up hungry. If the child awakens for another reason, the mother has a different response.

Take a few minutes to think about these examples. Ask yourself in each case how the information might have been transmitted. What is the common denominator? The answer is that we are beings of light—*every* living thing is. The electric processes of our body determine to the highest degree who we are, how our bodies work, and how they communicate with our immediate environments, the world, and the universe at large.

The current way of pursuing science and medicine is, in many ways, a dead end. Because the medical community believes that something is true only if it is scientifically proven and re-created, it loses one of the essential pillars that could be used for support: adjusting the treatment to fit the individual case, even when the treatment doesn't match up with the standard data. You can only compile a list of criteria for the "correct" treatment of an illness if you treat a human like a machine. The situation is as absurd as a 1910 manual titled *How to Repair a Car for all Times to Come.* Yet we are all individual cases, and it would be a blessing for a society to have more members with healing powers who are privy to this secret.

We sometimes run into people who argue that there is no room in modern medicine for the methods of our forebears. "Where would that lead us if we did that?" is what we occasionally hear. Well, we know it would lead to humane and cause-driven medicine. Of course it would create a few problems initially when integrating these methods, especially the Art of Timing—the timing of a multitude of daily activities in accordance with the lunar calendar and other natural rhythms. But that is not so important. What is important is that these methods are all valid and successful. For each treatment course and for each healing process, there are ideal times and also days when nothing can be achieved. This law of nature will not change, even if it creates problems, like making appointments in a hospital. What is most important is that a free society—a free mind—upholds the ability to decide freely the manner in which one finds and maintains optimum physical, spiritual, and emotional health.

We called the last section "Once Upon a Time," though we encourage you to rescue some of these strange leftovers from days gone by and bring them into our modern world. With them—and a renewed unity of spirit and mutual respect—we can build a good future for generations to come.

From around the age of six, I had the habit of sketching from life. I became an artist, and from fifty on, began producing works that won some reputation, but nothing I did before the age of seventy was worthy of attention. At seventy-three, I began to grasp the structures of birds and beasts, insects and fish, and of the way plants grow. If I go on trying, I will surely understand them still better by the time I am eighty-six, so that by ninety I will have penetrated to their essential nature. At one hundred, I may well have a positively divine understanding of them, while at one hundred and thirty, forty, or more, I will have reached the stage where every dot and every stroke I paint will be alive. May Heaven, that grants long life, give me the chance to prove that this is no lie.

Hokusai, Japanese painter

15

Rainbow Soup

A Birthday Wheel Elixir

We would like to show you a very practical yet simple use of the Code that invokes the spiral motion of the Wheel and the dynamic energy of the colors. We do not know of a better remedy for prevention and healing than our "soup of all colors," which our children call "Rainbow Soup." Even if you only accept this one recommendation from the entire book, namely, to indulge with your family in the blessings of this ancient medicinal-culinary recipe, you will have done more good for them than could ever be repaid in gold. This secret remedy is not only highly effective, but it is also extremely tasty. And though the recipe might appear complicated at first, after a while preparing it becomes second nature.

Ingredients
- A large pot with a tight-fitting lid
- A wooden spoon for stirring. No metal, no plastic!
- Vegetables, herbs, and spices in five colors: black/blue, green, red, yellow, and white. The selection of ingredients is left to your imagination and preferences. Celery root and salt (white), and parsley or lovage (green) are frequently used in Europe.

Preparation

1. First, divide the vegetables, herbs, and spices into five small piles according to color.
2. Clean the vegetables but do not peel them (especially if you're using onions!).
3. Next, cut the individual colored piles so that you get a few pieces per color. This is the only reason you have to cut up the vegetables.
4. Fill the pot two-thirds with cold water and put it on the stove on low. Now stir the water seven times clockwise with your wooden spoon. Why clockwise? Stirring clockwise generates energy, while stirring counterclockwise withdraws energy from any food or drink. The stirring should take about thirty seconds, about the time it takes to recite the Our Father, which is how they did it in Johanna's family (although you don't need to pray while doing it, just make sure it is done at least seven times).
5. Fill the pot with the vegetables, herbs, and spices using the following sequence:

   Blue/Black – Green – Red – Yellow – White and repeat
   Blue/Black – Green – Red – Yellow – White and and so on

Yellow can be added anywhere in the color sequence, but in our experience it is best after red.

Initially, add only a little of the first color pile of your choice to the pot—the color that you feel you need most. It is up to you which color you use first, but the ongoing sequence of colors must remain the same. For example, if you start with white, then black/blue must always follow.

After adding the first color, stir with a wooden spoon at least seven times clockwise. This will take about thirty seconds. Now add some of the next color. Stir again seven times or for thirty seconds. Add the next color and stir again, and so on.

Continue doing this at a leisurely pace until you have completed the color circle several times and no vegetables are left. The more often you complete the circle, the more medicinal the soup. It would also be a good idea to finish with the color that you or the patient requires in the current circumstance. Usually, the soup is already simmering when you get to the last color, and all the vegetables, herbs, and spices are in the pot.

Allow the soup to simmer covered for at least three hours. It is fine to do it in less time, but every extra hour intensifies the healing powers of the soup. In the case of a grave illness, the soup should simmer for seven hours on the stove.

Strain the soup and refrigerate for the whole week. Feel free to drink a portion immediately if you wish. (The strained vegetables will be a welcome addition to any compost pile.)

Additional hints for preparation of the healing-by-color soup

Preparation: Divide the piles of vegetables, herbs, and spices into bowls in the correct color sequence.

Black/Blue: With us, the black pile is always the smallest because we mostly use black peppercorns. (The white and the green piles are usually the largest.) The different amounts are not important, as it's all about personal preference and instinct.

Green: Lovage is important for the taste. Simply tear off a few leaves from the bunch or use a pinch of dried lovage. No lovage to be had? Parsley works, too. (You may want to order organic lovage online or start growing it in your garden for future use.)

Red: Chinese red dates from the Asian grocery are a favorite for us. We also use red peppercorns (which don't make the soup spicy hot) and red onions.

White: Root celery, onions, and leeks are all good choices, but use whatever you like or have available in the house. When white is called for, so is salt. Here you can also use rock salt, which has a pink tint, or Himalayan salt. Rock salt is always better than sea salt because of the state our oceans are in.

Yellow: Carrots, yellow beets, and yellow peppers offer excellent flavor and color, but again, go with whatever vegetables and seasonings you are drawn to.

Remember, there are no limits for your taste. Generally, you do not need additional spices, but the soup should taste good. Let your taste buds decide. And of course, use only organic products whenever possible.

How often should you eat this soup?

Have some soup every day, but only warm up as much as you need. Once you've tried it, you will not use bouillon cubes or stock packs again. This soup provides an ideal base for all sorts of tasty dishes. *Bon appétit!* And if you found the recipe beneficial, then don't forget to pass it on.

◆   ◆   ◆   ◆   ◆

In closing, we would like to remind you that the Birthday Wheel does not stand still—unless that is what you wish. The Wheel does not have blockages nor does it stagnate unless you choose for it to be that way out of fear or some other motivation. Nothing in the Code contains sentencing, judgment, or prejudice unless you judge or feed your prejudice with whatever fears lead you to it.

The Code is a tool that is meant to help and to heal. It is not meant to hinder you or to lull your mind to sleep. Accept it as a gift that will help you become and remain whole. Do it because you love yourself, and because you love life.

> *We need not continue living*
> *As we lived yesterday.*
> *Free yourself from this perception,*
> *And a thousand possibilities invite you to a new life*
> —**Christian Morgenstern**

Glossary

Birthday Wheel: The basic structure of the Birthday Wheel is used to determine your personal Code (of life gifts), and it always remains the same. Each direction of the compass—North, East, South, West, and Center—will always contain the same Numbers: **6** and **1** go into the North, **8** and **3** go into the East, **7** and **2** go into the South, **9** and **4** go into the West, and **0** and **5** go into the center.

Cardinal Points: North, East, South, West, and Center on the Birthday Wheel. They are occupied with Numbers from your Code, also known as Stations.

Center of Gravity: The Station in your personal Code with the most Units or weight/influence. The Center of Gravity is also affected by the last digit of your birth year, which holds more weight than the other Numbers in your Signature.

Code: The Code is what we call all aspects of this knowledge. Your personal Code comes from the four (minimum) to six (maximum) Numbers of your birthdate, excluding the century—month, day, and two-digit year of birth.

Compass: A shorthand drawing of the Birthday Wheel made with two intersecting, perpendicular lines.

Feminine Numbers: Numbers 6 through 0, which impart patience and thoughtfulness.

Linked Pair: A pair of two Numbers that occupy the same Cardinal Point and share the same color. There are five linked pairs.

Masculine Numbers: Numbers 1 through 5. These Numbers impart a fast-moving character, decisiveness, impatience, and recklessness.

Placeholder zero: These are zeros in a date that are not used for your Code. Only zeros in the tens column of the day number go into the Code, (zeros from the 10th, 20th, and 30th day of the month), and zeros in the tens column of the month, such that only the 10th month, October, contributes a zero to your Code (apart, of course, from year and decade).

Signature: Your Signature is made up of the Cardinal Points in which your Numbers are located—North, East, South, West, and Center. There are thirty-one Signatures in all.

Stations: The compass directions on the Birthday Wheel (North, East, South, West, and Center) when they are occupied with Numbers from a personal Code, also referred to as Cardinal Points.

Units: The weight or influence you have in a given Cardinal Point, determined simply by adding together the Numbers.

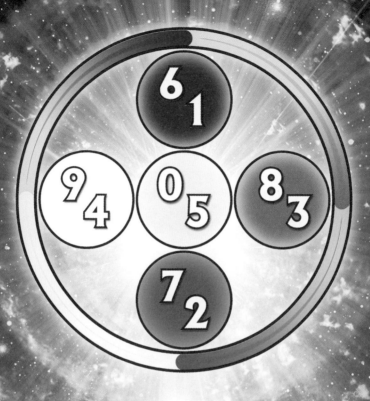

Numbers Chart

Birthdate Numbers	6 and 1	8 and 3	7 and 2	9 and 4	0 and 5
Zodiac Direction	North	East	South	West	Center
Color	Blue/Black	Green	Red	White	Yellow
Positive Aspects	Receptive Sensitive Intuitive Deep Thoughtful Gentle Visionary Determined Inquisitive Spiritual Courageous Wise Fearless Strong-willed	Nature-loving Uncomplicated Modest (when less than 10 units) Seeking harmony Hopeful Musical Compassionate Sympathetic Empathetic Patient Tolerant Creative Generous Selfless	Enthusiastic Lively, High-spirited Energetic Independent Economical Charismatic Being listened to Active Loves Change Passionate Joyful Inquisitive	Manually dexterous Religious Creative Industrious Enterprising Efficient Success-oriented Sharp-witted Assertive Cultivating good relations Successful Ambitious	Creative Willing to make sacrifices Generous Patient Nature-loving Balanced Centered Persevering Spiritual Sympathetic Caring Sensible Common-sensical Helpful Cooperative
Negative Aspects	Fanatical Annoying Harassing Burdening Easily offended Quickly bored Quickly irritated Indifferent Unenthusiastic Depressive Anxious Power-hungry	Manipulative Hairsplitting Destructive Intrusively curious Naive Gullible Stubborn to obstinate Spendthrift Irritable Easily frustrated	Tendency to overexertion Arrogant Haughty Domineering Revengeful Avaricious Quickly bored Erratic/volatile Tendency to extremes Tendency to exaggerate Greedy Mourning theatrically Tendency to hysteria	Contradictory Overly pedantic Deceitful Destructive Materialistic Ambitious Hypocritical Corrupt Unrealistic Greedy for power Calculating Egotistical	Squandering Distraught Dreamy Absent-minded Overly generous Overly permissive Tendency to pondering Tendency to fanaticism

Birthdate Numbers	**6** and **1**	**8** and **3**	**7** and **2**	**9** and **4**	**0** and **5**
Zodiac Direction	North	East	South	West	Center
Color	Blue/ Black	Green	Red	White	Yellow
Professions/ Areas of Proficiency	Innovator Pioneer Lawyer Thinker Author Diplomat Teacher Politician Judge Researcher Public Relations Public Media All Humane Disciplines	Healer Physician Nurse Psychologist Preacher Singer Musician Farmer Nursery School Teacher	Monk Revolutionary Priest (Preacher) Researcher Explorer Architect Philosopher Painter	Inventor Craftsman Technician Accountant Calculating merchant Mechanic Pilot Racecar Driver Athlete (out of ambition) Lawyer	Farmer Forester Horticulturist Politician Honest Merchant Geologist Patron Epitome of "Mother" Protector
Quality	Inspiration Willpower Depth Water Communi- cation (know- ledgeable)	Height New beginning Light	Temperament Proliferation Fire Wildfire Communi- cation (inspiring)	Matter Metal Tools Business sense Invention Crafts	Center Grounding Balancing of all extremes
Feminine/ Masculine Energy	Feminine **6** Masculine **1**	Feminine **8** Masculine **3**	Feminine **7** Masculine **2**	Feminine **9** Masculine **4**	Feminine **0** Masculine **5**

Note to Readers

If you would like to contact us, please send us an email at *vrz@aon.at*. We have also pitched our tents on the internet at *www.paungger-poppe.com*.

In addition to offering information about a variety of subjects, including excerpts from our books, our site provides a store, where you can order our books, calendars, and other products directly. Downloads of our Alpha/Omega questionnaires are also available.

Checking out *youtube.com* (search for "Paungger") will bring up "Life Lines—Johanna Paungger," a 45-minute documentary movie about us produced by a German television station, with an English voice-over. A great introduction to our work!

About the Authors

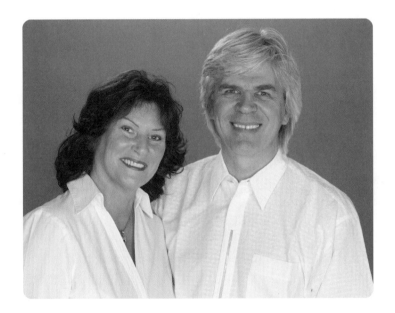

Johanna **Paungger-Poppe** was born and raised on a Tyrolean mountain farm in Austria. On this family farm, a special wisdom—now called the Code—was kept alive for centuries, and was handed down to Johanna in its entirety by her grandfather, a renowned healer and shaman by today's standards.

Author and translator **Thomas Poppe** published more than twenty nonfiction works on a variety of subjects—from alternative healing to

Eastern spirituality—before he met Johanna as a result of her search for a writer. For the next twenty years, Johanna and Thomas shared first an office and then a home, cowrote eight bestselling books and eight calendars, and became the happy parents of three children—with Thomas being unaware of Johanna's use of the Code in their daily routines all the while. Only her uncanny ability to remember hundreds of birthdates struck him as unusual, and eventually led Thomas to discover that she simply saw birthdates in full color and 3D in front of her mind's eye!

Through harmonious collaboration, a relationship where Johanna combined her knowledge and experience with Thomas's writing skills and expertise, this carefully guarded knowledge and terminology of the Code was reinvented and recorded for today, becoming an instant bestseller in Germany. Along with their successful writing careers, Thomas and Johanna operate a mail-order company, Der Mondversand, selling products such as natural cosmetics and herbal teas that are all developed around the principles given in their books and in accordance with the lunar cycles. Visit www.paungger-poppe.com to find more about their books, get advice on health, learn of upcoming author events, and get to know two of Europe's most successful nonfiction authors and how they are sharing their powerful knowledge with the world.

The Code Journal